Battlefield Surgeon

AMERICAN WARRIORS

Throughout the nation's history, numerous men and women of all ranks and branches of the US military have served their country with honor and distinction. During times of war and peace, there are individuals whose exemplary achievements embody the highest standards of the US armed forces. The aim of the American Warriors series is to examine the unique historical contributions of these individuals, whose legacies serve as enduring examples for soldiers and citizens alike. The series will promote a deeper and more comprehensive understanding of the US armed forces.

SERIES EDITOR: Roger Cirillo

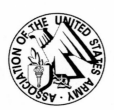

An AUSA Book

BATTLEFIELD SURGEON

Life and Death on the Front Lines of World War II

Paul A. Kennedy

Edited by Christopher B. Kennedy
Foreword by Rick Atkinson
Afterword by John T. Greenwood

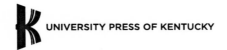

UNIVERSITY PRESS OF KENTUCKY

Scholarly publisher for the Commonwealth,
serving Bellarmine University, Berea College, Centre College of Kentucky, Eastern
Kentucky University, The Filson Historical Society, Georgetown College, Kentucky
Historical Society, Kentucky State University, Morehead State University, Murray
State University, Northern Kentucky University, Transylvania University, University
of Kentucky, University of Louisville,
and Western Kentucky University.
All rights reserved.

Editorial and Sales Offices: The University Press of Kentucky
663 South Limestone Street, Lexington, Kentucky 40508-4008
www.kentuckypress.com

All photographs are from the author's collection.

Library of Congress Cataloging-in-Publication Data

Names: Kennedy, Paul A., 1912–1993, author. | Kennedy, Christopher B., editor.
Title: Battlefield surgeon : life and death on the front lines of World War
    II / Paul A. Kennedy ; edited by Christopher B. Kennedy ; foreword by Rick
    Atkinson ; afterword by John T. Greenwood.
Other titles: Life and death on the front lines of World War II
Description: Lexington, Kentucky : The University Press of Kentucky, [2016] |
    Series: American warriors | Includes bibliographical references and index.
Identifiers: LCCN 2016006705| ISBN 9780813167237 (hardcover : alk. paper) |
    ISBN 9780813167244 (pdf) | ISBN 9780813167251 (epub)
Subjects: LCSH: Kennedy, Paul A., 1912–1993—Diaries. | United States. Army.
    Auxiliary Surgical Group, 2nd—Biography. | World War, 1939–1945—Medical
    care—United States. | Surgeons—United States—Biography. | United
    States. Army—Surgeons—Biography. | Surgery, Military—United
    States—Biography. | World War, 1939–1945—Campaigns—Africa, North. |
    World War, 1939–1945—Campaigns—Italy. | World War, 1939–1945—Personal
    narratives, American.
Classification: LCC D811.5 .K458 2016 | DDC 940.54/7573092—dc23
LC record available at http://lccn.loc.gov/2016006705

This book is printed on acid-free paper meeting the requirements of the American
National Standard for Permanence in Paper for Printed Library Materials.

Manufactured in the United States of America.

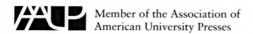 Member of the Association of
American University Presses

To my peerless father

To all the members of the Second Auxiliary Surgical Group

And, of course, to Ana

Contents

Foreword

A good diary can bring back the dead with a power denied even the most gifted physician. Paul A. Kennedy was an exceptional surgeon, but it is his journal of three years at war in North Africa, Italy, and western Europe that resurrects an era now more than seventy years gone. The story he tells, day by day, is vivid, poignant, and often shocking. Kennedy is as committed to his comrades and to his country's cause as any loyal soldier, yet the stark authenticity of his narrative makes this among the most compelling antiwar accounts of World War II.

As a proficient combat surgeon must, Kennedy works briskly through the long queue of broken soldiers who appear on his operating table— young men damaged by artillery, mines, gunshots, grenades, bombs, accidents. Through him we see entry wounds, exit wounds, transverse liver wounds, fractured skulls, amputations, gut perforations. Among the first battlefield cases he treats in Tunisia is an unexploded twenty-millimeter shell embedded in a soldier's elbow, not the sort of procedure normally taught in medical school. At Salerno, where he spends his first night ashore sleeping just beyond the beach, with only a towel for cover, he operates on an Italian boy who has lost both legs and an eye. "I never really knew until today," he writes, "what war means to civilians." The boy dies. On the Volturno River, he treats a soldier with "a piece of shell in his brain, a bullet in his belly, and his left hand blown off." Kennedy's skill as a draftsman in meticulously illustrating severe wounds makes his written descriptions even more wrenching.

Treating hundreds of combat wounded only enhances Kennedy's humanity. His admiration for ordinary GIs, particularly infantrymen, is unalloyed. "Arms and legs missing—dirty, foul-smelling wounds—and never a complaint from any of them," he writes. He mourns for widows who have yet to hear of their loss, like Ina Mae Warren of Iowa, whose corporal had "an arm and a leg blown off plus a thousand other wounds . . . So tonight, unknown to her, Ina Mae Warren is without her husband—and forever."

Like the army he serves, Kennedy becomes ever more adept as the war unfolds. Off duty, he studies surgery textbooks and seeks out experienced surgeons for advice. Through him we sense the brilliance of American technical skill, innovation, and logistical competence. Through him we also experience war's misery: mud, rain, bad food, incoming artillery, inconstant mail, air raids, loneliness ("an actual ache that I can feel"). He is an astute observer with a gift for evocative images. Aboard a troop transport bound for southern France, he puts in a shift as a watch officer down in a "dark hatch filled with sweating soldiers. Fortunate your sense of smell tires after a time and you smell nothing." During yet another artillery barrage in France he "hugged the earth with a fierce love."

A civilian at heart, he can be caustic about military life. "Hash, hash, beans, and more hash," he complains, then repeats the time-tested GI injunction: "Keep your mouth shut, bowels open, and don't volunteer for anything—that's the army." After an inspection by a senior medical officer, Kennedy writes, "He asked some awfully stupid questions for a guy who's supposed to be the boss of all medical installations." As a doctor who often lives and works in danger, close to the front, he disdains rear-echelon officers "all dressed up with their pants pressed."

War makes him acerbic. While treating wounded German prisoners, he muses, "We chase them like hell—shoot hell out of them—and then work like hell to keep them alive—for what?" In the best GI tradition, trenchant humor helps get through the day and through the war, as when he loses his dog tag and reflects, "I'll probably turn out to be the unknown soldier." Of an army bivouac in Algeria called Cactus Flats, he observes, "There's no cactus and it's not flat."

But the sure knowledge that what he does matters, that he is the difference between life and death for the next young soldier on his table, preserves Dr. Kennedy from cynicism. In the end, we come to know a man who kept faith with his family, his patients, and his country. This is a love story, written about those he saved and those he couldn't save. In these pages, they all live again.

Rick Atkinson

Preface

Military surgery is the surgery of trauma encountered in
epidemic proportions.
            —Edward D. Churchill, surgical consultant, ETOUSA

On November 2, 1942, my father, Paul Andrew Kennedy, sailed out
of New York Harbor on the *Santa Elena*. Bound for Casablanca, the
Santa Elena was part of the Western Task Force of Operation Torch, the
massive Allied invasion of North Africa. He didn't know this when he
embarked. He said good-bye to my mother at the gates of Camp Kilmer,
New Jersey, on October 31, wondering "where and why and home and
then you, Marion." Forty-eight hours out of New York, their destination
and mission were revealed to them.

Thus began what would be almost three years of foreign service, taking him to North Africa, Italy, France, Germany, and ultimately home
again to my mother and to the children he had left behind, Paul and Joan,
who were so young they could scarcely have remembered him. Also waiting for him was my sister Ruth, born after he left, whom he had never
seen.

He was a surgeon, a member of the Second Auxiliary Surgical Group.
After an initial period of relative inactivity in North Africa, he spent
most of his time in Italy, France, and Germany, working in field hospitals, which were mobile units set up immediately behind the front lines
to care for soldiers so desperately wounded that they could not be safely
transported back to evacuation hospitals. This was virtual battlefield surgery. Often working ahead of their own artillery, the Second "Aux" set
up mobile operating theaters, for the most part in tents, to care for griev-
ously wounded boys and young men, many of whom seemed to have no
chance of survival.

He was young, relatively inexperienced as a surgeon, and confronted
with medical cases of a level of seriousness and complexity that one would
rarely encounter in civilian practice. By the end of the war, he had meticulously documented 355 of these cases. For almost three years, he lived a

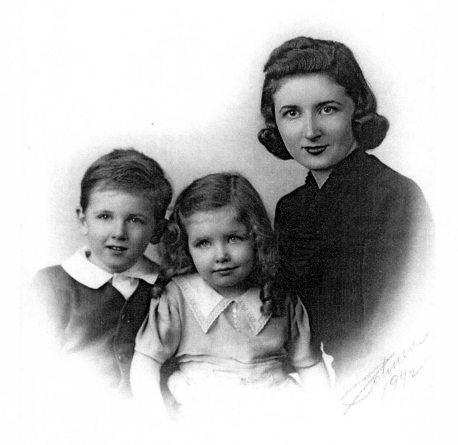

Paul, Joan, and Marion

kind of nomadic existence: he broke down, moved, set up, broke down, moved, set up . . . countless times, always keeping pace with the front. He saw Josephine Baker, George Patton, and Pope Pius XII. He lived underground among the troops pinned down at the Anzio beachhead while, as he said, German artillery, "the 'Anzio Express,' rode the wind." He entered Rome the day after it was liberated; he entered Dachau two days after it was captured by the Allies. He was uncomfortable, dirty, hot, cold, homesick, and most of all lonely. He missed my mother terribly; he longed to see his children. But the term of his service was indefinite. He knew he would return home only after the war ended.

Throughout his tour of duty he kept a personal diary, which was written for my mother. Starting in 1944, he also began to keep a clinical journal of surgical cases, which he illustrated. A talented photographer, he took more than a thousand pictures throughout his time abroad. What emerges from these documents and photographs is a full record of the experience of a medical officer in the European theater of operations in World War II.

Paul Andrew Kennedy was born on November 19, 1912, in Scranton, Pennsylvania, the third child and the older son of Martin and Mary Connor Kennedy. My grandfather took great pride in his children. He was an omnivorous clipper of newspaper articles and a compulsive saver of programs, letters, telegrams, and, indeed, any document, however insignificant, that he thought recorded and preserved the history of his family. These documents he kept in scrapbooks, which provide an oddly Kennedy-centric view of life in Scranton at the turn of the century and over the next forty years. Among all the dance cards, one-line telegrams, newspaper clippings, and programs from Knights of Columbus meetings, we can follow the thread of the early life of Paul Kennedy.

Scranton was at the time still essentially a mining town. It owed its existence in part to the beds of anthracite coal upon which it rested. Although its population surpassed 135,000 during the first thirty years of the twentieth century, study of my grandfather's newspaper clippings suggests that the city, racially and to a lesser degree ethnically homogenous, retained the quality of a small, insular town. In the *Scranton Times* we find, for example, an extremely serious-looking Paul Kennedy, high school winner of the Freshman Oratorical Contest. He poses stiffly, gazing somewhere over your left shoulder, in what appears to be quite a tight collar. There we find his exploits as the Central High School football hero, the outstanding quarterback in the area—not a great passer or runner but the clever caller of the unexpected play at the unexpected moment. We can follow him to Georgetown University as he wins the Dixon Medal for oratory, as he is named outstanding ROTC officer, as he plays quarterback for what was then a major college football program, eventually earning the nickname Little Thunder for his explosive barking of signals from under center. We see him clipped from the pages of the *New York Herald Tribune* as Georgetown prepares to play Manhattan at Ebbets Field. We discover that upon graduation from Georgetown he enrolled in St. Thomas College in Scranton in order to take the science classes necessary to apply to

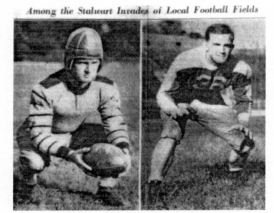

Among the Stalwart Invaders of Local Football Fields

New York Herald Tribune
article

medical school and that, while attending Jefferson Medical College, he married Marion Joan Haggarty, who was to be, as he put it, "my best and only friend" for fifty-six years.

After graduation from medical school in 1939, he began a year of internship followed by a year of residency in surgery at Geisinger Medical Center in Danville, Pennsylvania. He was called to active duty on July 20, 1941 and was assigned to the surgical service of Lovell General Hospital at Fort Devens, Massachusetts, where he served for thirteen months before being reassigned to the newly activated Second Auxiliary Surgical Group.

He was a young man of considerable—and varied—talents. He did, however, have his shortcomings. He was, for example, quite possibly the worst singer on the planet. It was only when I went to Georgetown myself that I learned that the various fight songs I had been listening to for years were not all to be intoned in a tuneless drone; they actually had identifiable melodies. Moreover, it is remarkable to anyone who knew him that on his army induction papers he claims some fluency in Spanish. As his diaries reveal, his ability to speak or understand any foreign language was, to put it charitably, limited. His assertions while in Italy that this or that situation was "no buono" reveal the extent of his facility with any language other than that spoken in Scranton. On the other hand, he was a superb athlete, a forceful speaker, a diligent student, and a talented artist.

Less readily apparent were the qualities that made him a gifted surgeon. He was meticulous, thorough, and invariably well prepared. He never undertook any task, however insignificant it might have seemed, without committing himself to it completely. Surgery for him was never the mere mechanical display of virtuosity; it was the first stage of a relationship with a patient. Indeed, the letters he received from recovering soldiers show evidence of his commitment to their welfare. Over and over they ask, "Do you care this much about all your patients?" He did. He never stopped caring in this way until the Parkinson's disease that eventually killed him forced his retirement.

His plan had been to fulfill his ROTC obligation with his year's service at Lovell. Events, however, proved to be more powerful than plans. As it turned out, he served more than four years. During that time he was, as the diaries reveal, miserable. To the pain of loneliness were added the physical discomforts attendant upon living for the most part in tents, and upon the nearly constant mobility that keeping up with the front demanded. He loved to eat, and the generally dreadful food was a real burden to him. Inactivity, particularly early in his foreign service, was nearly unbearable; he was not only separated from home, but he felt he was filling no useful role. Two things helped: mail and work. Mail was his only connection to all that he loved so much. He lived for letters from home, although, as he frequently said, they made him feel worse afterward. Work made the time go faster and it gave him a sense that all his sacrifice and unhappiness were in the service of useful ends.

Passing in and out of the life of this lonely, homesick surgeon were hundreds of wounded boys and young men. The difficulty of the task was daunting. The wounds he treated were disastrous; the boys for whom he

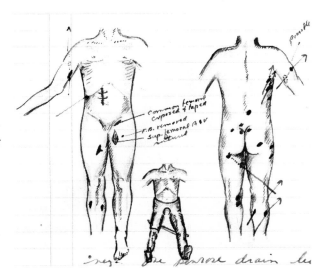

"He was completely wounded if a soldier ever was."

cared were maimed and mutilated. They came from all over the United States to find themselves thrust into a chthonic maelstrom of artillery shells, shrapnel fragments, mines, and bullets. There, in the cold lethality of modern war, they incurred the dreadful injuries that brought them to an operating table in some cold, muddy, makeshift field hospital and into the care of my father, who saved them.

I knew virtually no details of my father's service in World War II until after he died. Like so many veterans, he never spoke of it. So I was astounded to discover that he was in Operations Torch and Avalanche, that he had been at Anzio, that he landed on D-day in Operation Dragoon, that he had spent years in close proximity to the front lines, often under air or artillery bombardment. On those few occasions when I had asked him about it (and in retrospect, I was remarkably incurious), he replied only that he was "a doctor in the war." So he was, and to his mind, nothing more needed to be said. But his story is the story of all the members of his Second Auxiliary Surgical Group in the North African and European theaters of operations. There is, in fact, much more to be said, and I offer it here, mostly in his own words. Silent in life, here he speaks.

Editor's Note

Among the challenges of producing this book, perhaps the most difficult lay in finding the best way to integrate three disparate sources—diaries, medical journals, and photographs—into a unified, coherent narrative. The medical records meticulously detail 355 surgical procedures and include drawings of wounds as well as letters of gratitude from recovering soldiers. There are almost two thousand photographic negatives which, fortunately, my father carefully labeled. And there are the diaries themselves, originally in three volumes, one for each year of his service.

My initial intention was simply to transcribe the diaries and journals for my family's sake, and I pursued this in desultory fashion for a number of years. This was my great mistake: by the time I realized that there was an important story to be told here, that it deserved a wider audience, those who lived through the war years were gone, and their memories with them. I determined, nonetheless, that the materials at hand could be combined to make a significant contribution to medical military history and to the history of World War II.

The challenge, as I say, was how to do it. It wasn't until I had the negatives digitized and I understood how well the photographs could complement the diaries and medical journals that I began to see how the three sources could be effectively and engagingly interwoven.

The first step—editing the diaries—involved regularizing my father's sometimes capricious punctuation and use of abbreviations, silently correcting the most egregious misspellings, and also silently correcting errors of fact (for example, he refers to the "Baltic states" when he clearly means "Balkan"). In doing so, however, I also tried to preserve the unpolished immediacy of the diary form. In keeping with this idea, I did not correct his misspellings of place-names or add diacritical marks, particularly in the names of French and German cities. My original impulse was to correct all such errors and omissions, but I decided that to do so would not be true to the authenticity of the diaries.

Although my father wrote in his diary virtually every day for almost three years, the attentive reader will note that a number of dates are missing. In fact, I edited out about a quarter of the entries, particularly those from early in his service when even he says, "Sorry this diary is so uninteresting, but I'm not doing a thing so there's nothing to report." The aim was to convey his boredom without, at the same time, inducing it.

In choosing which entries to include, I tried to preserve those that portray his sense of the larger war, explicitly refer to surgical cases, and vividly convey what daily life was like for the members of the Second Auxiliary Surgical Group.

Selection of photographs was then guided by the narrative of the diaries. The exigencies of publishing, however, dictated that only about one-third of the photos I originally included could appear in the finished manuscript.

Inclusion of material from the medical journals also demanded finding a balance, this time between accurately portraying the surgical problems field doctors encountered while not overwhelming the general reader with technical terminology. While a trauma surgeon would find the details of operations interesting, I felt that a relatively small sample would suffice to depict what working in a field hospital entailed. To help the nonprofessional, I also developed a medical glossary. In doing so, I relied on my father's somewhat outdated medical dictionary (*Dorland's Illustrated Medical Dictionary*); I wanted to explain the terms as he would have used and understood them.

The reader who wants to see more of the photographs and surgical records will find them at the book's website: www.battlefieldsurgeon.com.

A number of entries make brief allusive reference to events in the war. Explanations of such references are included in the text in brackets.

Members of the Second Auxiliary Surgical Group are identified in brackets in the text of the diary and in the endnotes. I didn't feel that it was necessary to identify well-known public figures such as Montgomery or Patton. Many other individuals are named, some of whom can be identified, at least partially, by context; some, however, my father mentions without providing further information about their occupations or relationship to him. I would like to have provided complete information about every individual who appears in this record, but it simply wasn't possible.

My aim in producing this book was threefold: to convey the daunting challenges that personnel of the Second Auxiliary Surgical Group faced and overcame, to augment the scant historical record of frontline surgery in World War II, and to ensure that the memory of my father's goodness, dedication, and fundamental decency would never be lost "in the dark backward and abysm of time."

Introduction

The Development of the Field Hospital in the Mediterranean Theater

World War II shouldn't have surprised the United States—or the US Army—when it literally dropped out of the Hawaiian sky in December 1941. After all, it had been going on for two years by then. Nonetheless, if the arrival of war wasn't precisely a surprise, it certainly caught the nation—and the military—unprepared. This was particularly true of the Medical Department of the US Army: "American Military Medicine faced the crisis in an unpromising state—two small bureaucratic agencies serving the peacetime needs of the least impressive armed forces of all the major powers on earth." The plan for medical care in the field was—on paper—clear. A chain of evacuation of the wounded from the battlefield to the home front was envisioned, dependent on the establishment of a series of field medical units, but "short peacetime budgets meant that not much of this apparatus existed in reality."[1] In fact, at the beginning of the war, there were no mobile hospitals that could treat military personnel in the field.

As the Medical Department hastily developed infrastructure and augmented the ranks of medical personnel, it also had to develop protocols for caring for battle casualties that were suited to the type of warfare into which the army had been plunged. The lessons of World War I, with its largely static front lines, were going to have to be modified and adapted to the more fluid front lines of World War II.

In time, an effective evacuation system for treating battle casualties did evolve, especially out of the Allies' experience in North Africa and Italy in 1942–1943: "The Mediterranean Theater was able to write regulations that essentially set the pattern for front line medical practice in all theaters, including the Pacific." Colonel Edward D. Churchill, surgi-

1

cal consultant in the theater, later said that previous systems of combat medical care "were but faltering steps" toward the evacuation practices developed in the Mediterranean: "The whole basis of the chain of evacuation was echeloning . . . doing emergency work on the wounded at the front and more complicated work later at the rear."[2]

The concept of echeloning led to the development of the modern field hospital, mobile enough to keep up with the front but equipped with all the necessities of surgery. And in fact, the army field hospitals of World War II developed into nimble, adaptive units that "surpassed in flexibility any other hospital which the Medical Department had."[3]

A field hospital consisted of a headquarters and three hospital platoons, each of which could operate independently. Colonel Churchill insisted on the mobility of these units in the belief that the single most important factor in achieving a successful outcome for a battle casualty was to minimize the time elapsed between when the soldier was seriously wounded and when he reached the operating theater of a field hospital.

Churchill also observed in North Africa that communication among the links of the evacuation chain was poor and even at times nonexistent. A soldier might arrive at a clearing station without any indication of what treatment he had received in transit. To correct this, the system of "tagging" patients was developed. The initial point of the evacuation chain for a wounded soldier was the battalion aid station. The medics who manned the station attached a tag to the patient with his personal information and an indication of what, if any, treatment he had received. At each stage of the chain, the tag would be updated so that when the patient was admitted to the field hospital, the surgeons knew exactly what medications he had been given and how much plasma or blood he had received.

Each platoon of a field hospital was able to function independently as a hundred-bed hospital with its own personnel, transportation, and equipment. This independence allowed the platoons to "leapfrog" one another. Nontransportable casualties generally needed a week or so after surgery to recover before they could be sent back to an evacuation hospital. One platoon of a field hospital would stay in place as a holding company for these patients while the other platoons would move forward as the front moved. One of these latter platoons would then serve as the holding company while the one that had previously occupied that position jumped past it as the line moved again.

The field hospitals worked in concert with the medical battalion that was attached to each division. This battalion was made up of a headquarters, three collecting companies, and a casualty clearing company. The collecting stations, as the name implies, were primarily sites where wounded soldiers would be gathered from the battalion aid stations on their way to the clearing station, usually five to ten miles from the front.

Casualty clearing stations in turn served as the most forward hospital facilities. As such, they treated not only battle casualties but accident victims and personnel who had fallen ill. In the case of a soldier wounded in combat, the primary function of the clearing station was to evaluate the soldier's wounds and to determine whether he was stable enough to be transported to an evacuation hospital some fifteen to twenty miles farther behind the front. Alternatively, lightly wounded personnel could be treated and returned to the line. The most seriously wounded, deemed nontransportable, were sent as quickly as possible to a field hospital, which would be set up within litter-carrying distance of the clearing station.

The optimum physical configuration of the field hospital evolved as the war went on: "The receiving ward, shock ward, operating room, postoperative ward, X-Ray and laboratory form a cross. The receiving and shock ward is situated at the main entrance, the postoperative ward occupies the tent which is a prolongation of the shock tent, while X-Ray

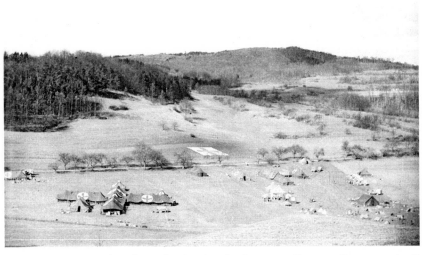

Tenth Field Hospital and 120th Clearing Station near Hausen, Germany, April 1945.

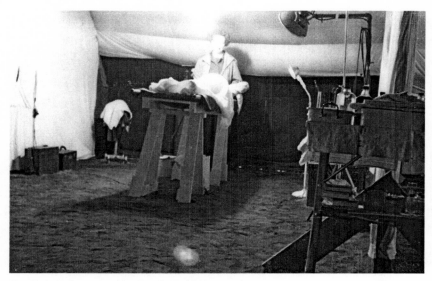

Operating theater at the Tenth Field Hospital.

and laboratory occupy a tent opposite to the operating room. A pyramidal tent forms the central point in the cross."[4]

Although field hospitals had their own medical personnel, the actual surgery was performed by teams of the auxiliary surgical groups (ASGs), independent units with their own headquarters, equipment, and transportation. Each "aux" team consisted of a chief surgeon, an assistant surgeon, an anesthetist, an operating room nurse, and two enlisted medical technicians. The headquarters of the ASGs determined where surgical teams were needed and assigned them accordingly. By late 1944, there were five complete auxiliary surgical groups, each comprising about twenty-five teams, in the European theater of operations.

This arrangement—the close and constant cooperation of fully independent field hospitals and auxiliary surgical teams—maximized mobility and flexibility, but it also occasionally created friction between the teams and the field hospitals in which they worked. The permanent staff of the hospitals performed routine medical procedures while the aux teams controlled the operating rooms (ORs) and performed all surgery. Moreover, the aux teams "had an aura of elitism and professional independence that set them apart." As a result, "auxiliary surgical group commanders devoted much effort and diplomacy to smoothing out these undercurrents of conflict."[5]

From the Battlefield to the Home Front: The Chain of Evacuation

Colonel Churchill is widely credited with refining the evacuation procedures that were so successful and so widely adopted in World War II. The stages of that procedure are well illustrated by the case of Stanley Levy, a nineteen-year-old private who was injured at 0700 hours on February 15, 1945, near Weismuller, Germany. He sustained gunshot wounds to the left forearm and abdomen. He was tagged at the battalion aid station at 0830 hours and given .5 gram of morphine sulfate. His arm was splinted at the 360th Collecting Company at 1030, and he reached the Tenth Field Hospital at 1100. His condition on admission was fair, with a blood pressure of 140/80. Over the course of the next two hours and forty-five minutes in the shock ward, he was given 500 cc of plasma, 1,000 cc of blood, and 20,000 units of penicillin. X-rays revealed a foreign body in an intraperitoneal position. He had also suffered a severe compound, comminuted fracture of the left ulna, involving the median, radial, and ulnar nerves. Examination of his left hand for function and sensation was unsatisfactory.

Surgery commenced at 1420 and lasted for more than two hours. The first stage was a laparotomy, which revealed considerable free blood in the abdomen. Eight perforations of the small bowel were closed and the foreign body—a machine-gun bullet—was removed from an intramesenteric position at the root of the mesentery at the ileum. The transverse mesocolon was perforated but the colon itself was intact. The abdomen was closed in layers and the entrance wound debrided. There was extensive destruction of the ulna and soft tissue of the left arm. The radial artery and vein were intact, but the median and radial nerves were destroyed. The wound was debrided and dressed with dry gauze and sulfa and a long arm plaster cast.

Private Levy's immediate post-operative course was uneventful, and he was evacuated in good condition on February 23.

In 2009, with the help of the Veterans Administration, I made contact with Mr. Levy, who was eager to talk about his experience and still grateful to my father after all those years. He wrote to describe his course of treatment after he was evacuated from the Tenth Field:

> In December 1945, I landed along with eleven other soldiers
> in my squad in Marseille, France. From there we began work-

ing our way up into Germany. My squad was a heavy weapons company bearing machine guns and mortars. Something that I remember distinctly is that it was very cold—five degrees. As we were advancing through the woods to the German lines, I got shot. A friend in my squad who was with me also got shot. When the blood hits the cold air, it steams, so you can't stay there because the Germans will aim at the steam. That is what we used to do. I figured I had to get out of there and get help because my friend who was wounded could not walk. I walked to an aid station and on the way there I remember that I almost passed out a few times from loss of blood. I remember that it was very cold but after walking for a while my feet began to get warm. When I got to the hospital, I realized that my boots were full of blood and that was why they were warm. When I got to the aid station they stabilized me, gave me fluids, and took me to a field hospital. That is where they operated for the first time. When I first got into the tent, one of the doctors was going to take my left arm off. When I heard this I raised hell. I was still awake and was not going to let them remove my arm. Your father intervened and said that he would work on me. When I woke up after surgery I realized that he had saved my arm.

I was there for about seven days before they moved me to the Thirty-Fifth Hospital—a regular hospital in Germany. I stayed there for about a month until I was well enough to be sent home on a hospital ship. When I got back to the States, I found that I had Hepatitis C from the blood transfusion I received in the field hospital. I was then sent to a hospital in Virginia where they treated me with glucose because that was the only treatment they had for that at that time. Then they sent me to Atlantic City because at that time the government had taken over all the hotels in Atlantic City, so I was sent there to recuperate. I was then sent to Hallern, Staten Island, New York. While there they took a bone graft and took a piece of bone from my leg and put it into my arm. I was also given a tendon transplant. All together, I think I had eleven operations on my arm during that time. I was at this hospital for about a year. After a year I was sent to a hospital in Valley Forge where I had scar evasion. All the operations were very painful. During this time my mother, my sisters, and my cousin would visit me often. In 1947 I was discharged and sent home to West Philadelphia from the hospital.

> After the war, I had trouble getting work because they would not hire disabled people and my left hand was paralyzed. So I started my own appliance business called Levy's Appliance. I was twenty-two. When I was twenty-three, I spotted a beautiful young lady at a restaurant in Philly called Harvey's. I finally worked up the nerve to ask her out and after about six months we were married. We had two sons, Jeff and Stan. In 1980 I retired and passed the business to my son Jeff.

The positive outcome for Private Levy rested on a number of factors, including the skill of the surgical team and the quality of post-operative care. But perhaps chief among those factors were the speed and efficiency of the evacuation process. He was evaluated and treated at the battalion aid station only a little more than an hour and a half after being wounded and was in a field hospital being prepped for surgery in only four hours.

Once developed and refined, this system of evacuation and forward surgery served the army well until the end of the conflict: "War surgery was the great lifesaver of those who were injured in combat, and in many ways the Mediterranean Theater became the army's teacher in the managing of the wounded. In staffing its hospitals with surgeons the theater . . . began with good material. The younger men at the forward hospitals were probably the best-trained generation of American surgeons yet to appear."[6]

They needed to be. Churchill likened the effect on the body of a high-velocity bullet or shrapnel fragment to "an internal explosion."[7] Wounded soldiers arrived at field hospitals "torn, shattered, and disemboweled, yet still alive. The wounds were ghastly to the eye and complex puzzles to the surgeon, who had to solve them quickly with lives hanging in the balance."[8]

The Surgeons: The Second Auxiliary Surgical Group

The Second Auxiliary Surgical Group was activated on April 10, 1942, at Lawson General Hospital in Atlanta. On October 6, in preparation for participation in Torch, the first detachment of eight general surgical teams (including Paul Kennedy), three orthopedic teams, and three shock teams was alerted. They left Lawson on October 8 for Camp Kilmer, New Jersey, where they were attached to the Eighth Evacuation Hospital. This small detachment boarded the *Santa Elena* on November 1 and sailed for

Casablanca in the early morning hours of November 2. The Second Aux arrived in the harbor on November 18, shortly after the armistice with the French had been signed, a group of surgical teams without nurses and without a headquarters, and therefore without consistent direction or organization. Moreover, "no formulated plans had been established for the proper functioning of an Auxiliary Surgical Group in this theater." They remained attached to the Eighth Evac, but "the casualties from the campaign had been light and the surgical teams were not needed."[9] They were to remain with the Eighth Evac for four months of almost complete inactivity.

Colonel Churchill, in the 1943 annual report of the consulting surgeon, described their experience in these first months:

> At the time of the initial landing and later during the early phases of the Tunisia campaign, the members of the Detachment of the 2nd Auxiliary Group were scattered here and there living the life of gypsies. There were no precedents that established their mission, no plans that defined the policies for forward surgery, and no adequate facilities for performing surgery in the combat area. These highly trained surgeons were transferred from one unit to another without explanation or designation of their function, bivouacked in pup-tents throughout months of cold and rainy weather and begged for transportation necessary to carry out urgent orders.

Finally, on February 27, 1943, the main body of the Second Aux sailed from New York on the *Andes* and arrived in Casablanca on March 9. Shortly thereafter, group headquarters were established in Rabat, almost immediately providing organization, coordination, and coherence to the mission of the surgical teams. In April, several teams were assigned to British general hospitals in Algiers, Bone, and Phillipeville, providing "the first opportunity for members of these teams to participate in the surgical management of battle casualties."[10]

By June, plans had been formulated to attach the Second Aux to Fifth and Seventh armies. It subsequently supported Seventh Army in Sicily and Fifth Army in mainland Italy, with teams landing on D-day in both invasions. By the time the Italian campaign was well under way, in the fall of 1943, the lessons of North Africa, Sicily, and Italy had been well learned and the Second Aux had begun to function as it would for the remainder of the war, remarkably smoothly and efficiently, considering the difficult circumstances under which it was asked to operate: "The entire unit was now together and functioning with a field Army on a mission for which it was originally designed."[11]

By the end of the war, officers of the Second Aux had treated more than twenty-two thousand nontransportable cases, had earned nine battle stars, and had received the Meritorious Service Unit Plaque. The unit plaque was awarded for actions in Italy in the fall of 1944, but it well describes the conduct of the entire outfit throughout the war:

The 2d Auxiliary Surgical Group is awarded the Meritorious Unit Service Plaque for superior performance of duty in the accomplishment of exceptionally difficult tasks. . . . Operating within enemy artillery range and under severe weather conditions, this unit displayed steadfast devotion to duty in the surgical management of the seriously wounded, greatly increasing the expectancy of survival by performing major surgery close to the field of battle. The unparalleled degree of technical skill and tireless energy of the personnel of the 2d Auxiliary Surgical Group resulted in the saving of countless lives of American and Allied Soldiers.[12]

1

Operation Torch and North Africa

Tuesday, October 27, 1942
Start

Should have started this sooner but at least started before leaving this country. Left Marion yesterday at 8:45 a.m. Please, God, bring me home safely to her and the kids—no matter the time. No idea as to our destination. Drew East India in the pool today but that is not the spot—I hope. Had final physical today. Weather good. T 50. Southerners wearing overcoats.

Heard rumor that restriction was to come off in a.m. Good news to sleep on.

Wednesday, October 28, 1942

Restriction off at 6 this morning. Called Marion and she arrived at 2 p.m. Staying at Kimel's—17 Graham St., New Brunswick, N.J. Very nice people—$1 per night. Drove to New York and saw *Strip for Action*—very funny. Ate at Rose's Restaurant on 51st St. Marion looking lovelier than ever—a remarkable girl. To bed at Kimel's at 12:30.

Thursday, October 29, 1942

No restriction on—means more time with Marion. Lunch at the diner—dinner out at Colonial Farms; all wives and officers. Rather a stupid gathering. Had four ryes and ginger ales before dinner—tasted unusually good. To bed at Kimel's at 11 p.m. Understand there is to be an alert in a.m.

Friday, October 30, 1942

Restriction on at reveille today was a mistake—were confined to post, however. Said goodbye to Marion at gate at 8:45 a.m. We said good-bye believing it wasn't the last.

Saturday, October 31, 1942

Restriction still on. Saw Marion at gate at 12:30 today. She looked pretty—was wearing her star. Told her I felt that this was our alert but she felt differently. Learned at 4:30 p.m. that we leave early in a.m.

Saw Marion again at 7 p.m. at gate. She was in good spirits and was lovelier than ever. Glad to have seen her so close to leaving. I had a million things to say to her but they all evaded me.

I honestly believe there is not another person in the whole world that can quite compare with Marion. I'm already looking forward to my return to her and the children.

Sunday, November 1, 1942

Left Camp K at 9 this morning by train. By ferry from B&O to Staten Island. Passed Statue of Liberty at 10:30 a.m. I'll be a happy fellow the next time I see that lady. Boarded *Santa Elena* at 12:30 at Pier 15 Staten Island.

Boat loaded to roof with troops of Services of Supply—but destination and purpose still a mystery. To be enlightened 48 hours out of New York. Food on boat excellent. Went to Mass at 4:30 p.m. Bunking in stateroom #19 on A deck. Nine officers in room. A million things have run through my mind today—where to and why and home and then you, Marion.

Monday, November 2, 1942

Sailed at 2:15 this morning with some 3,000 aboard. Dawn revealed us in the middle of a convoy of 35 ships—seven transports—12 destroyers—an airplane carrier, and one cruiser. Sea calm—weather perfect. Never saw so much water. Headed east-southeast. Breakfast at 7:45 a.m. Ate heavy. Spent morning watching convoy maneuver—zigzagging continuously. Fire drill and abandon ship drill in a.m. Light lunch at 11:45 a.m. Stomach perfect. Assigned to a first-aid station on promenade deck aft on port side. Have five enlisted men. I'm to run a dressing station there in case of emergency. Saw many fish running and jumping off starboard side this afternoon. Sat on sky deck with our group. Two of our boys sick. I'm tired tonight and believe I'll sleep. Late this afternoon we were heading almost due south. I think I like the sea.

Tuesday, November 3, 1942

Not much sleep last night—weather is changing toward hot side. Up at

6 a.m. to 6:30 Mass. Big breakfast—stomach still in good shape. Heard first guns this morning—pulse quickened. Ack-ack and some heavy guns from battleship *Arkansas* and airplane carrier. Sea running heavy today and ship has started to roll considerably. Course is still east-southeast.

Saw Marion Saturday night; three days ago—it seems like a million years ago. I'm lonesome. There's nothing to do but sit on the deck and think and watch the sea go by all day long.

Storm coming up tonight. Boat pitching and rolling fiercely—stomach feels queer.

Wednesday, November 4, 1942

Good night's sleep. Up at 7 a.m. Ship rolling badly. Making about eight–nine knots an hour as a tanker fell behind during night. Found at noon. Spent practically whole day below deck—raining, fog, and too much pitching to suit me. Stomach now undecided as to what it will do. Still eating all meals. Had another fire drill and two abandon ship drills.

At meeting of officers tonight mission of task force was revealed. We are a part of the Western Task Force whose purpose it is to take French Morocco. We are five days behind the attacking force which is supposed to land in and about Casablanca and take it. Force from England taking Algiers at same time. We are to land after the fireworks—should be about seven days from now. Believe I'm getting my sea legs.

[North Africa was at the time under the control of "Vichy France," the puppet regime that grew out of the French acceptance of the draconian terms of surrender imposed upon them by Hitler on June 25, 1940. The Wehrmacht had routed the French, overrun the north of the country, and would have captured or destroyed the British forces if not for their miraculous escape from the beaches of Dunkirk. Henri-Phillippe Pétain, hero of the battle of Verdun in the First World War and deputy to Prime Minister Paul Reynaud, assumed leadership of the French government on June 17. He immediately indicated his willingness to end the conflict and then remained as the virtually powerless prime minister of what was left of France.

Operation Torch was conceived as an alternative to a cross-channel invasion of Europe, for which the Allies were as yet unprepared. The operation entailed three task forces—the Western, Central, and Eastern. The Central and Eastern task forces sailed from England; the Western Task Force sailed directly from the United States to land in Casablanca. The targets of the Central and Eastern task forces were Algiers and Oran, respectively.

Meanwhile, the Allies had entered negotiations with Vichy French admiral Jean-François Darlan, Pétain's commander in chief, who fortuitously happened to be in Algiers on personal business. They convinced him of their overwhelming strength and the futility of resistance, leading him to declare an armistice—without Pétain's knowledge or approval—on November 8, ensuring the swift occupation of Morocco and Algeria.

The Germans responded with alacrity. By November 16, German troops had begun to arrive in Tunisia, moving westward to hold the line of the Atlas Mountains against the advancing Allied troops. There, they were to be joined by Field Marshal Erwin Rommel, who was fleeing westward after his defeat at El Alamein at the hands of Field Marshal Bernard Montgomery and the British Eighth Army, but who remained a formidable adversary. The battle-hardened Germans were to inflict stinging defeats on the green American II Corps at Faid and Kasserine Pass. Nevertheless, with Montgomery approaching from the east and the newly appointed General George Patton menacing them from the west, the outcome was inevitable. On May 13, when 275,000 Axis troops, their backs to the sea, surrendered at Cap Bon, the Axis presence in North Africa ended.

It was in North Africa that the Americans identified effective leaders and began to learn, at considerable cost, the art and the uses of modern warfare. There began the development of the military juggernaut that would, two years later, overwhelm the Wehrmacht in the west and crush it against the anvil of the Red Army.]

Thursday, November 5, 1942

Fourth day at sea with no unusual occurrences as yet. Weather continues to be rough and I'm sick of the ocean. Only water available for washing is salt water and it's impossible to make lather with it. My hair is stiff. Convoy is still intact and keeps formation with remarkable accuracy—nights are black as pitch. Fellow by name of Robertson [Robert W. Robertson, assistant general surgeon, later general surgeon][1] from Paducah, Kentucky, rooming with us and he keeps everyone in stitches.

Friday, November 6, 1942

I said earlier something about a heavy sea—I was wrong 'cause today it just about stood the boat on its ear—and a sailor called it "a little heavy." Dark all day and raining—the boat rolling so that at noon the dishes fell off our table. The waves reached higher than the boat at times. Other boats of convoy hardly visible all day. Rumor has it that we have four and a half more days to go but that doesn't sound reasonable. Did very little today but lie on my bunk—I have the lower of the three tiers. Everybody is sick of the sea and talk lots of their homes and families—I think of mine constantly!!

Sunday, November 8, 1942

A week ago today we embarked. Week has gone fairly fast in spite of all. Heavy wind today but sea calm. Supposedly we are 900 miles off the African coast—in submarine-infested waters and within reach of land bombers. Convey made a complete circle at 3 p.m. while destroyers met far to our west. One depth charge set off. Course due east-southeast then resumed. Positions to assume during air raid explained by ship's C.O. [commanding officer]. Understand ship has much ammunition in hold—nice thought. Most everyone is concerned about possibility of air attack and no one conceals the fact that they are scared.

Tuesday, November 10, 1942

Awoke this morning to find the sea perfectly calm—not even a ripple that a stone might make. Picture clouds plus a glorious sunrise made it a beautiful picture. Wrote to Mom and Dad saying I arrived safely—a trifle premature—but letters must be ready to go back as soon as we get there. At meeting of C.O.s it was learned—much to everyone's displeasure—that we would probably land this Friday. We all thought it was to be tomorrow. Ship's news suggests things going well but Casablanca is still in question. We feel it must have fallen by now—(maybe we'll have to turn around and go home). This boat is a hotbed of rumors. Heard rumor today that we were sunk yesterday.

Wednesday, November 11, 1942

Armistice Day—of another war. Had a real alert this morning. Plane spotted off to right of convoy and for a time it looked like a real attack. My battle station is on promenade deck rather high but has steel roof. Great relief to find it a friendly plane. Meeting of organization at 3 p.m. C.O. told us that fighting at Casablanca not going so good and that we'd probably have to stay out for several more days. Rumor also that two transport ships in first convoy lost by torpedoes.

Flash!! Radio news at 6 p.m. gave news of armistice at Casablanca—real armistice day for us. Most everyone believes we'll be there tomorrow.

Thursday, November 12, 1942

Disappointed today—no landing. Learned tonight that we have been 150 miles off coast of Casablanca all day. Don't know why we're stalling.

Had several alerts this morning but planes were identified as friendly. I'm getting rather used to this alert business. I automatically swing into a few prayers and an act of contrition. At 8:00 p.m. we got some suggestive news—dress for debarking was named. K rations for two days issued. We all packed our valpaks again, swearing that soon we were gonna throw half the stuff away. Mine still weighs a ton. Carrying two quarts of White Horse [scotch] in pockets of overcoat. Feel that morning will find us just off the harbor. I must say that I'll be happy to set my feet on firm soil once again. I'm thankful to God for a safe passage.

Friday, November 13, 1942

Again we rode in circles all day. Within 75 miles of land. Harbor supposedly is full of ships, rumor has it. Ocean quite rough—new moon and evenings getting brighter. I'm getting awfully sick of being on this ship and so is everybody else. If we stay out much longer, a sub is gonna get one of us. Laid on my bunk most of the day thinking of home, Marion, and the kids and the wonderful year we had together in Groton.

Sunday, November 15, 1942

Third Sunday on board and still without any idea when we're going to land. Somebody did some bad figuring. Spent most of the day on the boat deck. My stomach and legs have become quite accustomed to the sea but I'm still anxious to get off and feel land under my feet. One fellow in the room, Larry Hurt [Lawrence E. Hurt, general surgeon],[2] is scared to death and talks constantly of landing. Drew Robertson's picture today and it turned out nicely. Immediately, all the group wanted their portraits—I've got some work on my hands.

Monday, November 16, 1942

Still aboard ship doing some fancy wandering. We go south all day, then north all night. Somebody said they saw land today but nobody else could find it.

Drew several pictures today. I'm swamped with requests. Keeps me busy, which is something. Had charge of calisthenics this afternoon and really gave the boys a workout. Trouble is we got all sweated up and then can't take a bath. Drinking water is even being rationed at this point. There is no bathing water at all except salt water and that's worse than nothing.

Tuesday, November 17, 1942

Awoke to find us still at sea in more ways than one. Rain chased the sun all day—traveling east. New moon waxing—sky tonight is brilliant—ships plainly visible. Pretty definite now that we're going in. Two battleships joined us tonight. All guns are loaded for first time. I feel good tonight and much relieved. Sooner things happen, sooner I'll get home. I love my wife and children.

Wednesday, November 18, 1942

Land!!

(1) 12:00 noon

Somebody awakened me at 3 a.m. to say they could see lights on land. Didn't sleep much after that. Mass at 6:30. Thanked God for safe, uneventful journey. Sighted land at 9:00 a.m. along port side of boat; everybody quite elated, including myself. At 11:00 a.m. we began to pull into harbor. Sun bright and very hot; ocean real green. Land was very green. Looks like big city from boat. Everybody looking for zebras, lions, etc.

(2) 2:30 p.m.

As we closed in on the harbor our convoy strung out single file—we were fourth in line. Harbor itself shows no damage of attack but French warships and transports badly damaged. Two French battleships half sunk and badly damaged. Four or five destroyers sunk and damaged. Five transports sunk. One of our freighters had big torpedo hole in side but wasn't listing. Casablanca from ship seems to be a modern city. Palm trees looked pretty to me.

(3) 12 midnight

On board ship. Spent most of the afternoon on boat deck watching other ships of convoy dock. French tugs did a good job. We're all bunched together, forming a nice target for planes.

Rumors are rampant again. We supposedly lost six ships in the action here. Also there is sniping going on in the city. 12 soldiers were shot last night. (I'll stay home nights.)

Africa—the name has always meant things so very far away. I never thought I'd see any part of it. I'm over 3,100 miles from home but my heart is with you, Marion.

Thursday, November 19, 1942

Happy birthday—this was probably the most eventful birthday excepting the first one that I have ever had. Got off the boat at 3 p.m. and carried our full packs and valpacks, a total of 150 pounds, about a mile. Our valpacks were collected then and we proceeded to march five miles to an

Italian school which had been vacated. We walked through the center of Casablanca and got a first look at the place.

Ate our K rations for the first time. They consisted of a can of ham, several hardtack biscuits, and a bar of chocolate. Some of the boys had gotten some red wine and we drank that. It was the best in the store and costs about 25¢ in American money. I didn't like it much. There are four hospital units housed here at the present time. No equipment of any kind as yet so we're sleeping tonight right on the concrete floor. I'm gonna take a Nembutal capsule, otherwise I won't sleep. Several units are going out tomorrow and I sorta hope we clear here. I'm anxious to see some work.

I'm tired tonight and think I'll sleep. I don't feel too badly—yes, I'm lonesome, but I know Mom and Dad are thinking of me on my birthday. And Marion has thought of me all day—cried a little, too, perhaps. She's awfully sincere in her tears. I love her.

Friday, November 20, 1942

First full day in Casablanca. Little better situated but not much so. We're still in our classroom sleeping on the floor. Strange as it seems, I slept fairly well last night. Up at 8:00 this morning and ate my K ration. Had dried biscuits and coffee and a fruit bar, plus lots of water. We're drinking water that we brought with us.

I led the calisthenics at 10:00 a.m. That's to be my job from now. Ate another K ration at noon, which consisted mainly of cheese and dried biscuits. Had powdered lemon to make lemonade—it wasn't bad. Went on a march at 2:00 and got caught in a driving rainstorm—everyone got drenched. Went to town at 4:00. It's a strange place indeed. It's modern and it isn't. The shops aren't well kept and the eating places are few and far between. We had several glasses of beer in a sidewalk cafe. Cost 2 francs a glass. Had dinner, which consisted of brown bread—no butter— soup (onion, I think), cauliflower, and ravioli. Not good but better than K rations. Had red wine with our meal, no water.

We were told today that we could write letters now and say where we are. I'll write in the morning. We are without lights here. I'm writing this by flashlight. It's now 8:30 p.m.

Saturday, November 21, 1942

Had a miserable night. This floor is getting harder and I'm getting less sleep. No signs of getting out of here yet. Had a K ration breakfast but couldn't get hot water for the coffee powder—drank it cold. Had calisthenics at 10:00 for an hour. They're calling me superman 'cause I'm a little strenuous. Went for a march at 11:00 and walked for an hour. We rather like the marches 'cause we see the town. Ate another K ration for lunch which was mostly cheese plus a little lemon juice. We're out of rations right now so we're hoping they're gonna start a kitchen soon. Bathing facilities are nil so I'm still washing out of my helmet. I actually took a bath out of it this afternoon and felt pretty clean afterward.

Wednesday, November 25, 1942

Nothing new today except that footlockers arrived and so I got my radio. Got England—sounds good; maybe later we can get U.S.

Started messing with the 8th [Evacuation Hospital] today—same food but it tastes better when you don't have to cook it. No more news about moving out. Sorta anxious to get going.

One of the boys just came in with four bottles of champagne. We drank to Thanksgiving with a hope we'd be home next year.

Thursday, November 26, 1942

Thanksgiving Day—Had a real Thanksgiving Day dinner—no turkey but rather roast beef—it was real good. Did nothing else all day except to write to Marion and to repack my footlocker.

8th Evac has hospital fairly well set up. 25 ambulances brought in many patients today. Few fractures in walking calipers but not much else.

No news about leaving.

All of group rather quiet today. Lonesome. Last year we had a good Thanksgiving—had two, in fact. I hope that next year we're back together—Marion, my lovely wife, and Paulie and Joanie (weather cool today).

Saturday, November 28, 1942

Second Saturday in Casablanca and it seemed like the longest day of the year—didn't do a solitary thing but walk a little bit. I'm getting awfully tired of waiting for something to happen.

We haven't been away from the U.S. long but everyone is wishing we were back. Somebody's always asking what you'd give to be home—to spend a weekend with your wife—I feel the same—I'd pay an awful price.

Sunday, November 29, 1942

Moved again to new quarters and to another school—a Jewish school this time. They're all the same, not one of them has a bed in it. We're still sleeping on the concrete floor and my back is awfully sore. Tomorrow I'm gonna find a cot if I have to look all over Casablanca.

We're near the ocean now—about six blocks away. Walked down tonight as we had heard that our convoy was pulling out. We saw it just as it was going down over the horizon—empty. Going home only 100 and some miles away from my loves. I've been lonesome since I left but something broke when I saw them. Oh, Marion, I miss you—sometimes I almost despair—but I don't—I know—I'm sure I'll get home. I love you, darling.

Tuesday, December 1, 1942

Went down to the docks today in search of a cot but could find none. Saw the *Jean Bart* at close hand. It had two large holes in it—one in the bow and a large one in the stern. It was a brand new battleship but now it's ruined. There was a lot more damage done along the decks than I had previously seen. The air corps and navy certainly did some accurate shooting.

Wednesday, December 2, 1942

I've got a pretty rotten cold in my head. I'm all stuffed up—damn sleeping on the floor—but it's all over now. Went down to the docks today and went aboard a freighter—the *John Mitchell*—and talked a navy ensign into giving us four cots—so now I'm off the floor for good. The ensign, Mr. King, was on a transport that went down off Labrador. They say in the U.S. that no transports have been lost—I know of several to date. I guess it's best that they keep such things quiet.

Friday, December 4, 1942

Worked in the dispensary of the 8th Evac Hospital today and was kept quite busy—saw 24 cases. It seemed good working with patients again. Mail was distributed today but in small amounts. I wasn't among the lucky ones. Now I have to wait until about Christmas before I hear. I'm certainly glad Auntie gave me my presents before I left. I'll at least have some Christmas. Supposedly a convoy will arrive here D40, which is December 20—I'm hoping it carries my Christmas. I've got plans to keep busy on the 25th 'cause it's going to be a particularly hard day to get by.

My radio is working swell now. Heard Lord Haw-Haw tonight. He certainly sounds like an Englishman but he talks like a German.

[William Joyce, the American-born fascist living in England, rose to the position of director of propaganda in the British Union of Fascists in the 1930s. In 1939, believing he was about to be interned by British authorities, he fled to Nazi Germany. There he recorded propaganda broadcasts for the English Service of German radio, chiefly aimed at the United Kingdom, where he came to be known as Lord Haw-Haw. Shortly after his final broadcast on April 30, 1945, he was captured by the British and charged with treason. He was executed in January 1946.]

Papers and some radio comments are talking about the war ending in 1943—Let's hope so.

Monday, December 7, 1942

A change in the weather—it was a real August day—sun shining and nice and warm. Played ball this afternoon and had quite a crowd watching us. I banged my finger and tonight it's quite swollen. Had all my surgical instruments out this morning and went over them with my enlisted men. It felt good to handle them again—makes you sort of anxious to get doing something.

The 8th opened up another little hospital today near us and two of our men are running it. It's to be a convalescent place. They're overloaded with patients now. They're gonna need a general hospital here very soon.

Tuesday, December 8, 1942

Another day gone by. For all the good I've done in North Africa so far I might as well be in North America. This business of just sitting around is getting on my nerves and everyone else's. They evidently expected lots of work right here in Casablanca and didn't get it.

Heard today that next convoy is coming in here December 18 so maybe we will have mail before Christmas—I hope so or Christmas will be a real bust!!

Wednesday, December 9, 1942

Three meals and a ballgame which I umpired constitute December 9th's activity. I'm spending a good portion of time reading my *Surgery of Modern Warfare*—the books I bought in New York. Every man has some surgical book and they're all different so we have quite a library.

Saturday, December 19, 1942

Got my first letter from Marion today so I'm feeling pretty good. I must admit that when I read it I was as nervous as a cat and I almost cried real tears. It was letter no. 2 so there is a no. 1 missing. I immediately sat down and wrote a long one in return. Worked in the hospital annex all day as O.D. [officer of the day]—not very busy—wrote letter to Marion and one to Reeve [Reeve H. Betts, thoracic surgeon], Gordon [Gordon F. Madding, general surgeon], and Leigh [Leigh K. Haynes, assistant general surgeon, later general surgeon][3] at Lawson. I wonder where they are now.

Less than a week now until Christmas—and not a sign of Christmas anywhere around—maybe next year!!

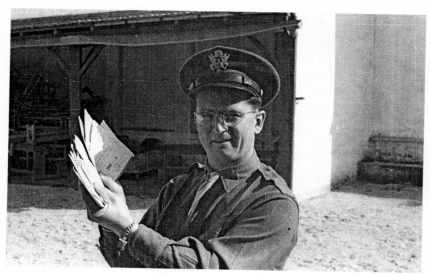

Mail!

Wednesday, December 23, 1942

Christmas party called off today. Convoy not in as yet so we'll have no meat—let alone turkey. I guess I'll survive but a little something extra on the 25th would help. That's how wrong it is to build and look for a Christmas of purely temporary gifts. A real good Christian should find this as happy a Christmas as any.

Had a V-mail[4] from Dad today dated December 1st—it was a good letter—I liked what he said about Marion and the kids.

Rode out to the airport on my bike with Taylor [Floyd D. Taylor, assistant general surgeon, later general surgeon]. They have given a considerable number of P40s to the French—the Lafayette Escadrille squadron is here—of World War I fame. Saw some B17s. Lots of big transport planes out there. Talked with some of the men that have bombed Tunis. They're all real young—and have what it takes!!

Thursday, December 24, 1942

Christmas Eve—and it's a pretty lonely one. I'd give the world if I could only be home tonight—even if it was only for a little while. Oh, Marion, how I miss you tonight.

Convoy of 10 ships came in at noon—so soon I should have some mail and presents—probably about Monday. I'm looking forward to your gift, Marion. (There are a lot of things I'm not going to be when I get home but the chief thing that I promise never to be again is selfish. We're without, and without a lot, and I guess in a way it's a good thing. It's easiest to understand the other fellow's slant when you've seen it from close hand.) God willing, I hope I'm home next year—if not, I'll make it the following year!!

Friday, December 25, 1942

Christmas Day—no different from any other Casablanca day. Warm sun shining brightly. Went to 9:00 Mass. Army chaplain read it at Sacred Heart Church. Opened Auntie's two presents and enjoyed very much that little bit of Christmas. Have received no mail or Christmas packages. Got lousy dinner—meat loaf.

Sunday, December 27, 1942

Meals are still all out of cans. Hash, hash, beans, and more hash.

Tuesday, December 29, 1942

Meals are absolutely lousy now. The mess officer has no imagination whatsoever. I never saw so much canned stuff in all my life. It's so long now since we had fresh meat that I doubt if any exists.

No mail from Marion.

Sorry, Marion, this diary is so uninteresting but I'm not doing a thing so there's nothing to report.

Thursday, December 31, 1942

New Year's Eve—and we're celebrating it by expecting another air raid. Last night at 3 a.m. we were awakened by antiaircraft fire and then by the sound of planes. Got our tin hats on quickly and then we stood outside (like nuts) watching tracers make flaming streaks across the sky. Flash lites lit the sky from all around the city and kept waving powerful beams back and forth. Five enemy planes went over—frequently they were caught in the searchlight beam. They were low enough to see the swastika on their underwings. Antiaircraft batteries put up an awful stream of fire. One four-motor bomber was hit—we saw it. It flopped over and later fell in the sea. I've read for months about air raids, what they're like and so forth, and now I know. It was really a wonderful sight. I kept repeating the act of contrition. I was afraid, I guess, 'cause I was shaking. It lasted from 3 a.m. until 5:30 a.m. Today I collected a few pieces of shrapnel. I'll save them. I hope God will see me safely through all. I hope he helps me do my duty.

Sunday, January 3, 1943

Slept through breakfast again—missed pancakes, too. 9:30 Mass at Sacred Heart Church.

Four teams got orders to go to Oran by motor, thence east by sea. Probably headed for Algiers. C.O. asked for volunteers but none were forthcoming. Keep your mouth shut, bowels open, and don't volunteer for anything—that's the army.

Wednesday, January 6, 1943

I don't think any group of men, particularly doctors, ever spent a more useless existence than the one we are spending. We do absolutely nothing all day long. It gives you so much time to be lonesome in. General Patton talked to all group commanders today in very harsh tones, saying that "we'd be meeting" the Germans any morning now and if the men were as poorly disciplined as the officers we'd be in a "helluva fix." Patton is all blood and thunder.

Bolton [Bernard Bolton, assistant orthopedic surgeon][5] told me today that he's sure he's gonna crack up. He's always in the dumps.

Wednesday, January 13, 1943

The 2nd Surgical Group split again today—10 men left by train for Constantine—56 miles west of Bizerte. They traveled in day coaches which were the typical European type. Had two boxcars same as used in World War I (40 men and eight horses). Now only 23 of us left here. According to reports we're to go out very soon.

No mail today. I'm disgusted with the mail situation.

Sunday, January 24, 1943

As I read back over some of what I've written, it seems rather foolish to record it all. I do so much of nothing.

Wednesday, January 27, 1943

My Xmas

Got three Christmas packages today—Mom and Dad, Auntie and Uncle Jack, and Marion. Marion's and the kids' pictures are beautiful—can't keep my eyes off them.

News of conference out—W.C., F.D.R., combined chiefs of staff of U.S. and England here for 10 days starting January 14. At Anfa Hotel. Suspected that F.D.R. and W.C. were here days ago. Conference biggest of any such war gathering—all concerned pleased with outcome. I'll be pleased if I come out—alive.

[The Casablanca Conference, headed by Winston Churchill, Franklin D. Roosevelt, and their chiefs of staff, had two notable outcomes: it was decided that, upon the successful completion of the North Africa campaign, Allied troops would proceed to invade Sicily; it was also determined that the only terms that the Allies would offer to, or accept from, the Axis would be those of unconditional surrender.]

Thursday, January 28, 1943

Today I really hit the proverbial jackpot—got 18 letters and a good number from Marion. It's pretty hard to place the letters chronologically—some are so old, others fairly recent. Marion, Ruth, Dad, Mom, Auntie, Uncle Jack, and Dad and Mom H. are all faithful correspondents.

From their letters it sounds as if war is beginning to pinch the U.S. By the end of this year, they'll really feel it. Nothing new here.

Monday, February 1, 1943

Heard rumor that Sicily had been invaded by British yesterday. Last of Germans before Stalingrad have fallen. Watching carefully what they do in Caucasus.

[The German defeat at Stalingrad was a catastrophe for the Axis powers, involving, as it did, the destruction or capture of the entire Sixth Army and the first surrender in history of a German field marshal. With this victory, the initiative on the eastern front passed irreversibly to the Soviets, who were not to relinquish it until they raised the Hammer and Sickle above the crumbled and smoldering ruins of Berlin.]

Saturday, February 6, 1943

Had some information today that the rest of the 2nd Auxiliary is coming in either on the next convoy or the one following it. Met a lieutenant colonel in Marrakech that had just come from Algiers. He told us of the terrific bombings they had had three nights in a row. Poor Russell [Alexander F. Russell, general surgeon][6] will be scared to death.

Opened some of Auntie's Xmas box and had some wine with it—Bolton and I. All tasted pretty good. Still just sitting but now there are very few complaints—everybody is reduced to the vegetable kingdom and is resigned.

Monday, February 8, 1943

The mail situation is fast becoming lousy again. Haven't had mail in a dog's age. And I'm very anxious to know if there is to be another addition to the P. A. Kennedy family.

Have taken up checkers at this point. Wish I'd get a letter from Marion—oh, how I miss her. If only this damn war would end.

Saturday, February 13, 1943

Finally got a letter—a V-mail from Auntie written February 2—pretty fast. But still no letter from Marion. Sometimes I feel like I am absolutely lost here—so lonesome all the time. Everybody is the same but I always feel that none of the rest have half as much at home as I have—they're not missing half as much.

Bolton being sent home—on a psychiatric diagnosis. Believe it is the correct thing to do but some of the outfit resent it. Calling him yellow—this comes from a few stupid individuals.

Monday, February 15, 1943

Two V-mails from Mom today (February 3). Why is the post office so efficient at slowing the wives' mail?

I was thinking tonight how absurd this whole situation is—here I am on a strange continent miles from home—sitting doing nothing, supposedly fighting a war—and mad at nobody in particular—except perhaps the mailman. If you ever stop to be rational about this whole thing you're lost. You'll immediately begin to lose whatever little grip you might have previously had on yourself. Fighting in Tunisia is heavy—yesterday Germans drove 18 miles into Allies' position west of Sfax. No word of today's activities.

Tuesday, February 16, 1943

Kharkov fell today and I'll fall tomorrow if I don't get a letter from Marion. It's like going without food to go without mail from my darling wife.

Heavy fighting in Tunisia. I would say that reports suggest Germans are besting it.

Headquarters suggested to Russell today that we're gonna be in demand shortly. I'm sure no one is anxious to get any closer than we are—!! I think I'll be damned scared but I won't be afraid.

Wednesday, February 17, 1943

News of fighting on part of Tunisian front not so good. German armored troops have now pushed 35 miles into American-held territory—about 80–90 miles west of coast between Sfax and Sincre. Heavy American casualties reported.

I actually have a real desire to get near the front—if I'm ever to do any good here it is now.

Thursday, February 18, 1943

Big event of the day was six letters from home—two of them from Marion. This is the first word I've had definitely that Marion is pregnant. I'm really happy about it and I know Marion is too. I wish I could be home with her through it.

Fighting on central Tunisian front has ceased. Believe they have taken all the ground they want and will now consolidate their positions.

Had a beautiful picture of kids from Dad today—Joanie is a beauty. I'm sure her *sister* will be too.

Monday, February 22, 1943

Benny left this morning for the boat. To sail on the *Argentina*. There is great to-do about him. Some few persist in making it unpleasant—calling Benny yellow.

He's carrying several gifts and a letter to Marion for me. Is gonna call Marion when he gets home.

Now I'm alone in the room.

Tuesday, February 23, 1943

Was down to the docks today aboard the *Argentina*—to see Benny. Boy, how I would have liked to stay right with her. I'd like to be going home, but not like Benny is.

Had little lunch tonight in Robertson's room. Everybody chips in— cheese, crackers, anchovies, sardines, Auntie's fruitcake, and hot chocolate (from D rations). We all gather in one room to listen to B.B.C. news at 9 p.m. and then sorta plan the war—and somehow we always get around to talking about when we'll get home. Some nights it's an early return—sometimes it's years.

Wednesday, February 24, 1943

Germans meeting stiffer resistance on central Tunisian front. Column heading toward Thala was thrown back to within three miles of the Kasserine Pass. Radio has not mentioned much of the bombings on Europe—hope they haven't slowed up because of losses.

Thursday, February 25, 1943

News from central Tunisia much better. Germans tonight are withdrawing through Kasserine Pass.

Played volleyball this afternoon—laid in sun. Hard life. This kind of an existence is much harder than if we were working.

No mail.

Friday, February 26, 1943

Am arising these mornings about 9 a.m. Have coffee and dry toast in Robby's [Robertson's] room—usually discuss the war in general and set a new date for its end. Much bitching today—fellows are getting letters from home telling of promotion of their friends.

Heard today from Casablanca billeting officer that a place near Anfa is being made ready for the 2nd Auxiliary Surgical Group—March 15 they're expected.

News from Tunisia all good now. I'd like to be near there. Will welcome orders to move.

(I love you, Marion, very much.)

Sunday, February 28, 1943

Radio tonight told of new German offensive in northern Tunisia along a 70-mile front repulsed at all points. Kasserine Feriani recaptured. Total war casualties to date in war is 66,000.

From the looks of things now I'm sure that we're headed for victory but it's gonna take too much time. I was looking at Marion's and the kids' pictures tonight and honestly, I felt like crying. How can a man be so lonesome?

Monday, March 1, 1943

Today marks my fourth month on foreign duty—seems more like four years. Will I ever get home to Marion and the kids?

Took charge of annex today—place has been in an awful mess—too many bosses. I'll at least clean it up. Colonel McKoan [John W. McKoan Jr., commanding officer, Eighth Evacuation Hospital] inspected this afternoon and was quite pleased with the improvement.

Still no mail from Marion—tomorrow, surely.

Tuesday, March 2, 1943

8th Evacuation got orders today. They pull out in a week. We are to stay, so our association formed in Kilmer is to end in Casablanca. 6th General Hospital to take over all patients.

Warm today but rained off and on.

No mail from Marion.

Berlin raided last night—8,000-pound bombs dropped (19 bombers lost). Fighting in Tunisia has been all favorable. Expect 8th Army to start this week—rumor says.

Wednesday, March 3, 1943

Rumors are again flying—we are evidently going into the field this weekend. Colonel McKoan returning from H.Q. Says that he got it rather straight that we're going "up." About time. We supposedly are now attached to 5th Army under General Clark. They're getting ready for something. If the Germans are as confused as we are, they must be in a stew.

Thursday, March 4, 1943

Hottest day we've had so far: 82 in the sun. Learned today that we are to move with the 8th—probably by tomorrow we'll not be going. Hate to give up these excellent quarters but actually I'd like to get going.

Rzhev captured by Russians—Germans routed. This is a serious blow to Hitler. Rail line from Leningrad to Moscow now clear and the pistol pointed at Moscow has been unloaded.

From all reports the trigger is about cocked in Tunisia. All lost ground in central Tunisia has been retaken.

Friday, March 5, 1943

We learned today that an unescorted transport is expected on Sunday—carrying 6,000 troops and rest of 2nd. They're to be billeted temporarily in a replacement pool near Fedala—40 miles from here. Question whether we'll join them or not.

No mail—oh, how I'd love to go home. Sometimes I get discouraged—it's hard to see any end to this thing. I love you, Marion, and miss you always.

Saturday, March 6, 1943

Large freight convoy came in today but no transport. 2nd due tomorrow. Played softball this afternoon—in shorts in March. It's hard to believe that this isn't summer. Most everybody out somewhere tonight—Robby and I here alone. This has gotten to be a very trying situation—can you imagine doing nothing—absolutely nothing for four months—going no place—just sitting and thinking—just sitting most of the time.

All this time I could have been home with my wonderful family. I have been useless so far here.

I'm so cockeyed lonesome that I'm half sick all the time.

Tuesday, March 9, 1943

2nd Surgical arrived today on unescorted transport. 90-some officers, 150 enlisted men, and 80 nurses.

Saw Leigh and Gordon—Gordon is now a major. My chances for promotion here are nil. I think I'll take the first chance I get to get out of this "bastard" outfit—that's what it's been—nobody wants us.

Had supper with Leigh and Jarvis [Fred J. Jarvis, general surgeon] and Munslow [Ralph A. Munslow, neurosurgeon][7] at Petite Poucet tonight. They were all full of questions about things to which I didn't have the answer.

All very enthusiastic—ready to go, etc.—so am I—ready to go—home!

Wednesday, March 10, 1943

We had a letter from Major Frank [Norris H. Frank, anesthetist][8] today—he went out in January. They're right up on the Tunisian front working in a clearing station, sleeping in pup tents, eating British rations—being strafed—not good.

Saw Major Betts today. He's living out at Anfa for the present. That's a beautiful place. Took several pictures from the roof. Had dinner with Gordon today. He's certainly an extrovert—he's thinking of nothing now except the nurses they brought with them.

We were reassigned today to our own group and start messing with them tomorrow. Colonel Forsee [James H. Forsee, commanding officer, Second Auxiliary Surgical Group] out here today—he doesn't impress me as being very forceful.

Had November and December mail today—nice, huh?

Friday, March 12, 1943

Major Park [chief surgeon on Kennedy's first team] had E.K.G. today—he's got signs of an anxiety neurosis. It won't surprise me a great deal if he is among the missing soon—who I'll get for a chief I don't know.

Saturday, March 13, 1943

Lost a dog tag today—now I'll probably turn out to be the unknown soldier.

Saw a pretty good movie tonight—one of Ann Sheridan's early ones—what a woman!! Rumor—better than that—we're actually going to move to Rabat—in tents—probably this week.

Major Park talked with Colonel Forsee tonight about himself—result, he's to have complete cardiac checkup at 6th Evac. He is physically unsuited for this type of unit but there is also present a definite anxiety—I can smell it!!

Monday, March 14, 1943

Orders requesting one team came in tonight—our team up next but no decision on Major Park yet so we're side tracked—Russell to get it. He doesn't want to go and is making every effort to get out. Robby hates like hell to go out with Russell. This is certainly a "screwed-up" organization. We were certainly shortchanged on the promotions. Merit doesn't seem to have anything to do with it, so it's not worrying me—too much.

Wednesday, March 17, 1943

Broke into the mail column today—letter from Ruth dated March 4—last one from Marion dated February 9.

Heard a lieutenant colonel in the air corps tell about blunders made in Faid Pass in central Tunisia in February. 1st Armored Division practically wiped out—lost 100 tanks in 40 minutes of fighting. Americans failed to defend either side of high ground above the pass. Patton made lieutenant general and sent recently to this command.

Hoeflich [Werner F. A. Hoeflich, anesthetist][9] got orders today—he's going to Tunisia. That is the beginning of a breakup of our team. Now I'll probably be peeled off. Just as well to get rid of Park. We'll see what time does!!

Friday, March 19, 1943

Heard a lieutenant colonel just returning from Tunisia talk tonight to the entire 2nd. We knew most of what he had to say but he took the wind out of some of the new bunch. They all believe themselves to be a group of high-powered specialists—what the war needs is some good general doctors who can do without and still get along.

Sunday, March 21, 1943

Received general absolution today—went to Communion—asking that God keep Marion safe for me.

Dan Dougherty [Daniel V. Dougherty, shock team][10] came back from Tunisia tonight and told us of his experiences. Left here in early January—to Constantine—joined 9th Evac, then to 51st Medical Battalion. Worked in clearing station and did real surgery. Was in Gafsa just before Germans came in. Withdrew to Kasserine Pass, then had to evacuate that place. He has been in the midst of the war. Our other men acquitting themselves well, he says. No news on our moving today. Enlisted men and nurses gone.

Monday, March 22, 1943

Some of group moved to Rabat today—we are supposed to move tomorrow. I have felt lousy ever since I got Marion's letter this evening. A letter should make me feel pretty good but it made me awfully lonesome tonight. I have no idea when I'm gonna see her again. When I think it may be a year—perhaps two—the thought almost kills me.

Tuesday, March 23, 1943

Suddenly got word this morning that we were going to move. Packing gently reminded me that I still have much too much stuff. Two trucks required to move us. We took everything that wasn't nailed down—chairs, tables, and everything. Rode in an open truck to a place just outside Rabat—some 60 miles from Casablanca. Camp set up on a racetrack. 11th Evac right near us. Four captains to a tent—three majors. I'm living with Larry Hurt, Leigh H., and Ralph Munslow. Tents old squad type and so are crowded. First meal we had here was good—steak from the U.S. No lights except candlelight so to bed early after 9:00 news.

No letter to you tonight, Marion, will have to do my letter writing in the daytime—but I love you, darling.

Wednesday, March 24, 1943

Had a poor first night in my tent. The wind blew a mile a minute all night and I was sure the darn tent was gonna blow away. Raining all night and continued throughout the day. I think I got wet a thousand times.

Spent the day trying to arrange things in my corner of the tent. The meal situation is definitely not good. Raining like hell and you have to stand in line in the rain and then eat it in the rain—like a picnic in a teeming rain. Had to evacuate my lower sigmoid—no cover on the eight-holer—sat in a drowning rain and was practically flushed into oblivion.

Friday, March 26, 1943

Raining again most of day—always at mealtime so I got at least three soakings.

I used to think I was lonesome for you, Marion—I thought I couldn't be more lonesome. But I was wrong. Oh, darling, I miss you more than ever. I love you, Marion, with all my heart—I always will until there is no more me.

Wednesday, March 31, 1943

Two letters today but none from Marion. I figured it out today—I'm getting 44% of her mail. Not a good score for Uncle Sam.

Gordon's team, plus a few others, was alerted today. What they're gonna do with us is a question—I have the poor major hanging around my neck like the proverbial millstone. Poor fellow is really scared to death.

Beautiful weather now—hot sunny days. I'm getting a real tan.

Monday, April 5, 1943

Foggy most of morning but sun out bright and hot this afternoon.

Had group calisthenics and road march—we're back to that kind of stuff.

Went into Rabat this afternoon and took a shower at the Red Cross. Finally got a pair of pants at the cleaners—not my own, but at least they're pants.

Robby got Russell's team. Munslow, neurosurgeon, given a general team along with Shefts [Lawrence M. Shefts, thoracic surgeon].[11] Much bitching.

Wednesday, April 7, 1943

Had a very fitful sleep—dreamed of Marion and the kids then I kept waking up feeling so lonely. I thought maybe I'd get used to this but I miss Marion more every day—miss her in a thousand ways.

Calisthenics and road march this morning. Played ball this afternoon, then exercised and ran around the one-and-a-quarter racetrack.

Munslow and I have a "Joy thru Health Club." I'm in pretty good shape right now.

Had long debate in tent tonight with Munslow and Haynes on what makes a man face fire.

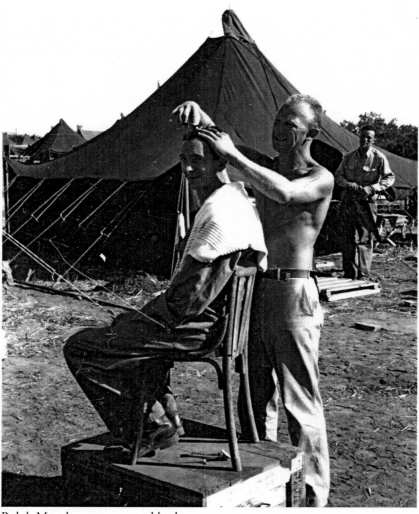

Ralph Munslow, surgeon and barber.

Thursday, April 8, 1943

Another red-letter day—got six letters but they were not of very recent vintage. Two from Marion—oh, how I long to be back with her—what a great day that's going to be.

General Patton's army has now joined up with the 8th Army. The air fighting, according to all reports, has been heavy and is very much in favor of the Allies.

I'm ready to go home right now—I sometimes wonder if I'll ever make it.

Saturday, April 10, 1943

News on the radio tonight was good—Sfax fell this morning and Rommel is still running. Americans pressing east at Fondouk threatening Rommel's flank. Boys all enthused and optimism runs high. Home by Christmas stuff is prevalent—but I doubt.

Had a real athletic day—baseball, once around the track, and then touch football. I'm really in good shape.

Tuesday, April 13, 1943

12 general surgical teams alerted today—supposedly going to Tunisia. Again old Park wasn't on the list. I'm afraid I'm not going to see any part of this war. Maybe I don't know when I'm well off—this way at least I'll get home safely and that should be my only concern.

Still doing nothing—calisthenics, road marches, and a few odd things. Seems like a terrific waste of time. Maybe in the end things will all add up to mean something worthwhile.

Wednesday, April 14, 1943

Another great day for the mail—got 14 today plus a *Saturday Evening Post* of April 3. What a whale of a difference just a few letters made. The stories they tell me of the kids' doings make me lonesome. I'm missing one of the best periods of their lives. As long as I get back to them I'll be happy.

Read Marion's letters again before I got in bed—she's one girl in a million and she's all mine—what a lucky guy I am.

Saturday, April 17, 1943

Have lights now but the darn things are so dim I'm still writing and reading at night by candle.

The colonel told Park that he was assigning an anesthetist to our team so we would be ready to go.

Saw a movie tonight at Red Cross—Sonja Henie—sandwich and coffee afterward. Radio reporting 24-hour bombing over Europe.

Tuesday, April 20, 1943

Had two letters written in April today. The mail is certainly improving and will get even better.

(Someday something interesting is gonna happen and I'll have something to write—until then this will be a dreary recording.)

Attended a buffet supper that Tony Emmi [Anthony J. Emmi, shock team][12] gave for the officers in celebration of the birth of a daughter. Had a good time. Hope I have a daughter too.

Thursday, April 22, 1943

One of teams recently returned from the front demonstrated the application of the "Tobruk" splint—plaster and a Thomas splint.

Started taking Atabrine [an antimalarial prophylaxis] today. Two grams biweekly—will take this up to and through November.

Had a formal Retreat this evening. This place is getting like a C.M.T.C. [Citizens' Military Training Camp] more every day.

Saw a good stage show at Red Cross tonight. Josephine Baker.

Friday, April 23, 1943

Received first photographed V-mail today written April 12. Auntie in her letter said Marion was getting awfully big—could it be twins!!

Got news today of the execution by the Japs of the flyers who bombed Tokyo last year—makes my blood boil to think of it. If they're not made to pay for it, it will be a crime.

No sign of any work yet—just sitting playing soldier. Still some teams alerted. I still carry the major on a string around my neck. I'll probably end up in the Old Soldiers' Home.

Thursday, April 29, 1943

Mail from Marion and Auntie—always a good day when I get mail.

Atabrine day and what a day. We had a casualty list of 50, 20 of which had to be hospitalized. I got sick to my stomach and vomited everything I ever ate. Hope I don't repeat next Monday. Medical meeting tonight. Gordon M. talked on burns—did nicely.

Progress in Tunisia slow but steady.

Friday, April 30, 1943

We're moving—had it once removed from the colonel that we're going some place that takes five days by truck—in all probability Algiers. I feel certain that an invasion is gonna take place in June—just hope I'm not in that first wave 'cause somebody's gonna get hurt. Two letters today—one from Marion. I love her—miss her constantly.

Stomach still on blink—butterfly feeling.

Sunday, May 2, 1943

Our team is alerted—nurses still attached so we must be going to a British general hospital. Only waiting on moving orders now. It's been a long sit—six months—but now we'll finally see some work. I doubt, however, if it will be much. This is only a temporary thing before the invasion. Had hopes of teaming up with Gordon but I guess that's out for a while.

Rain here all day—miserable and cold—hope it lifts 'cause I won't like flying in soup.

Monday, May 3, 1943

Still awaiting orders—colonel most secretive fellow I ever met. It seems the entire organization is gonna move Wednesday. Have all my stuff ready to go. Boys tied one on in the tent tonight. Gave Leigh my fifth of scotch and quart of rum to get rid of it. Gordon got drunk, Leigh higher than a kite. Leone Poole [Harold L. Poole, general surgeon], Bill Bowers [Frederick W. Bowers, anesthetist], Charlie Dowman [Charles E. Dowman, neurosurgeon], and Lyman Brewer [Lyman A. Brewer III, thoracic surgeon].[13] Munslow came in in the middle of it plastered. I had to lead Gordon home—he was funny (in case it isn't clear, I didn't have a drink).

Had a grasshopper invasion here today—thousands of them as big as birds. We were batting them around with clubs.

Tuesday, May 4, 1943

We're leaving here at 4:30 a.m. by truck for Casablanca, from there by 7:45 a.m. plane to Oran and on to Algiers. We're going to the 96th British General Hospital, which is just seven miles out of Algiers. Miss Campo [Amanda R. Campo, nurse], Lieutenant Schneiderman [Benjamin I. Schneiderman, anesthetist], Major Park, and I—Delorey [George A. Delorey, surgical technician] and Clark [George W. Clark, surgical technician][14] the enlisted men.

Somehow I don't look forward to the air ride but it's better than the trains they have here. Main Group is gonna move to Oran either tomorrow or the next day. Letter today from Marion. (How I miss her—and need her, too!!)

Wednesday, May 5, 1943

Up at 4 a.m. to Casa by truck and then by 7:45 plane (*Dry Run*) to Oran. Arrived there at 11:30 a.m. Had very smooth ride—took several pictures from the air. Left Oran in *Dry Run* at 12:30 and landed in Algiers at 2:30. By truck out to Mason Caree, which is seven and a half miles from town. British General 96th Hospital there. We're sent into Algiers, where they (96th) have a 150-bed convalescent hospital set up in a French civilian hospital.

Thursday, May 6, 1943

My "batman" [a member of the staff of the British 96th General] awakened me this a.m. and presented me with a steaming cup of tea. Breakfast at 8—more tea. Schneiderman and I each have a ward—Captain Burns (British) has the third ward. Major Park to oversee the cases. At present time place filled with convalescents from Mason Caree. Tea again at 11— and tea for dinner at 1. Tea at 4 and more tea at 7:30 dinner.

Wednesday, May 12, 1943

Rather a dull day—changed a few casts—but the dullness of the day is frequently quickly relieved by the coming of evening. At 9:30 the air raid siren blew—I was in hospital as M.O. [medical officer]. 10 minutes later the guns started blasting away, making more noise than I ever dreamed could be made. We're in a bomb alley three-quarters of a mile from the docks—a premature release of bombs has several times razed the houses about where we are. Saw one plane go down in flames. Not so many lights here as in Casa. Half hour after the raid shrapnel wounds started coming in—worked 'til 2 a.m. Raid on for two hours.

Thursday, May 13, 1943

Took a Cook's tour this afternoon through the Casbah, the native quarter, and was amazed at the sights. I took many pictures—one I took as we walked through the prostitute section—the three gals in the door shrieked and ducked in the house. Thought I'd be knifed—felt good to get out.

Uncle Gerald paid us another visit. The heaviest barrage yet was thrown up—the buildings shook, glass broke all around—saw four planes go down in flames. I think you could get used to these things. Casualties were quite heavy—worked 'til 5 a.m. Took a 20-mm navy shell—which hadn't exploded—out of an elbow. One laparotomy.

Friday, May 14, 1943

Tired as can be tonight—I'm going to turn in as soon as I finish this page. Learned 50 bombers were over last night. Damage to docks and shipping was slight—the port is filled at present. Two hospital ships—British— were in at the time.

Monday, May 17, 1943

Three letters today but all old—April 4. Nice long one from Marion, with letters from Paulie and Joanie enclosed. They're growing up so fast I'll never know them. Gosh, I'd give anything to be with them.

Hospital is slow now and will be, I guess—the source is cut off, of course. Believe we'll get out of here in a few weeks

Wednesday, May 26, 1943

The radio is beaming forth with "There Are Such Things"—from B.B.C. (I don't believe it.)

Amputated a fellow's leg today—he got his foot caught in a loop of heavy rope which was suddenly pulled taut as a freighter pulled out. Fellow was 17 years old. Got in 60 patients this afternoon—mostly old cases. Some of them had been German prisoners—they were treated very good, they say—got good medical care.

I'm awfully lonesome—I'd give a million dollars to be home with Marion now—more if I had it 'cause she's worth a lot more!

Thursday, May 27, 1943

Miss Campo had a letter from Madding today in which he said that he understood we'd all be together soon—might mean we're going back.

Have them sleeping on the floor in my ward now but there's nothing to be done for any of them. Most of the wounds in are caused by mortar shells and land mines. Have one fellow who is on the verge of dying—he said to one of the sisters that he was glad he was going home now—his wife had just had a baby. Nice—huh?

Saturday, May 29, 1943

Rather busy all day. Redressings are quite an extended procedure and require an anesthetic as a rule. It really hurts to see some of these boys— the way they've been shot up—arms and legs missing—dirty, foul-smelling wounds—and never a complaint from any of them. We'll be seeing them on the streets of the world for years to come. It seems to me that they almost pay a greater price than the fellows who are killed outright.

Sunday, May 30, 1943

Did three big dressings this morning, which consumed the whole forenoon. One kid had had a gas infection and had recovered but his leg is useless now. Some of these wounds are terrific.

Friday, June 4, 1943

Slow day but busy night. Major P. [Park] and I went over to Special Service headquarters to a show and in the middle of it the air raid siren blew and we blew for home. We didn't quite make it, so the last few blocks in the rain of shrapnel was a little thrilling. Watched the raid from the hospital roof and it was quite a sight. The rockets have a weird sound. A bomb fell half mile from us, and it sounded as if it had hit us. Had 20-some casualties in. One an American sailor in bad shape. His gun got hot and blew up. To bed by 3:30 a.m.

Tuesday, June 8, 1943

Red-letter day again—22 of them—from February 12 to May 17—that covers the field. Napoleon was wrong—an army travels on its mail. Colonel Forsee in town—some radical change going on. He dropped in on us for five minutes and said teams are being shuffled. Major Park to see Colonel Churchill tomorrow. This may be my chance to get off #6. 3rd also being shifted around, so the colonel says.

Wednesday, June 9, 1943

Major spent a few minutes with Colonel Churchill today and I gather from their conversation they have something cooked up for the major—probably his exitus from the 2nd Surgical. Colonel Forsee said that all teams were about to be called back and rearranged. Hope I get on with someone decent.

Very warm here today—just baking.

Friday, June 11, 1943

M.O. again today so a little more busy than usual—the regular run of lacerations but one good amputation. That hand case I did is recovering nicely from his compression paralysis—had me worried for a bit.

Pantelleria surrendered this morning at 10:00. Sicily must be the next stop. Wrote a batch of letters to the family today. I should write more often but writing once a week to everyone is quite a bit.

Tuesday, June 15, 1943

Orders out today—we're leaving here by train Thursday at 5 p.m. for Oran. All but two orthopedic teams will be with us. I'm looking forward to leaving this place.

Nothing new here—hospital is full but dead—all cases merely waiting evacuation and so nothing to do for them. I believe that in a short time I'll be making up for all my inactivity.

Wednesday, June 16, 1943

All clear at hospital and set to leave tomorrow. They say they're sorry to see us go and I believe they mean it. It's been interesting meeting some Britishers at close hand—working and living with them. Gives you an opportunity to really get to know them. We judge too harshly 'cause we always put ourselves up as the norm.

I have every hope that my association with the major is at an end—I think it will be.

Thursday, June 17, 1943

Said good-bye to all at Mustapha after tea today then went to headquarters for supper. Then to station in Algiers. Train made up of three third-class coaches and some 10 boxcars—old 40 and 8 cars. Train left at 8:30 p.m. Seven officers in our compartment and piled in the car were American, French, and British soldiers plus a lot of Zouave [French light infantry] troops. No place to stretch out so Brinker [Herbert J. Brinker, general surgeon][15] and I got out and ran up along the train to our boxcar. Tried to sleep on the baggage but it was no use. Next to the engine and no springs, so back to our car. I climbed up in a luggage rack but this was useless. Got a few winks sitting up but mostly I just sweated out the night. Train going about 15–20 miles per hour plus long stops.

Friday, June 18, 1943

Starting and stopping all day and the sun blistering hot—we're inland just on the edge of the desert and there's no sea breeze. C rations for our meals plus some tea the British made periodically. Natives quickly gather at every stop begging candy and chewing gum. Are these our brothers in the flesh?—dirty filthy people.

Land we're riding thru is cultivated and appears fertile. Hay fields,

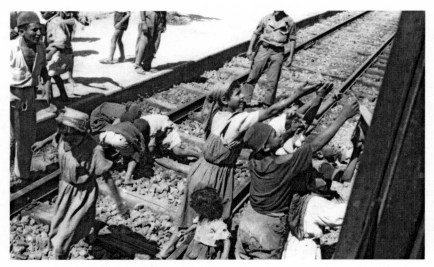

Beggars at a train stop between Casablanca and Oran.

great vineyards, olive groves, and some apricot trees. Very picturesque country—took several pictures. My eyes closing all day for want of sleep and always very thirsty—water we had was queer. Stopped in tunnel once for 10 minutes—thought I'd suffocate—but didn't, you see. At midnight we're 27 miles from Oran.

Saturday, June 19, 1943

Arrived in Oran at 3:30 a.m. Lights on in station—looked good. To Ain-el-Turk, where headquarters are by truck just 10 miles west of Oran. Got a cot and was asleep in nothing flat. Up for a good breakfast of eggs at 7:30, feeling fit. What a difference in the food. Campsite is a good one set on a little bluff overlooking the Med [Mediterranean]. Mess hall pleasant, well screened off and quite clean. Swim at 11:30 with Madding and again all afternoon. Nice beach at foot of Company St.

Seven teams have left for invasion group. Madding was to go, with me as assistant if I got back in time—but I didn't. Perhaps it's a good thing. Russell again in command so it will again be all screwed up. This is a nice place—hope we stay here for a few weeks.

Monday, June 21, 1943

Still haven't got the habit of this diary—I always seem to forget it until I'm well in bed.

Major Park going in hospital again tomorrow and then is to be transferred out of this outfit—colonel told him today. So my days with the
major are over—good!

Thursday, June 24, 1943

Got word at noon today that we're on the move again—probably Monday and we're headed for Tunisia—somewhere near Constantine. I knew
this place was too good to last.

Schneiderman gave a party tonight in honor of his new baby. All the
old gang gathered in one bunch to sing songs. We had a good bunch in
that original crew.

Friday, June 25, 1943

Up early this morning 'cause I had to pack my things before breakfast.
My bedding roll is still too big. Finally got away from Ain-el-Turk at 10
a.m. in a weapons carrier. Baggage piled on in all directions. Drove to
Bon Hanifin, about 60 miles inland. Natural hot springs where a French
spa was built—21st General set up there in great style. Had lunch, then
to 128th P.O.W. camp at Tizi. Large camp out on a dusty plain. 14,000
prisoners. They are herded together like cows but look awfully healthy.
I couldn't help but feel sorry for them. Back to Bon Hanifin for supper.
Then a good hot bath and to bed.

Monday, June 28, 1943

Up at 6:30 and started our chase all over Algiers in search of a million
different units. Finished our inspection at 5 and immediately drove out
to El Biar to the 95th General British. Had dinner there with John Adams
[John E. Adams, orthopedic surgeon] and George Donaghy [George E.
Donaghy, anesthetist].[16]

After dinner we drove out to the area where our teams who are in the
invasion group were camped. Found them all gone but Glenn Summers,
who is now attached to the 16th combat team. He was a lonesome soul
and was glad to see us. Rest of teams are already aboard ship and have
left Algiers. Summers says they all might be going to Tunis. I think it's just
as well that I'm not in this group of commandos.

Thursday, July 1, 1943

Finally had to go and join the group—got out to the 79th Station—just
past Fort D'lean this morning. Only half the group had come up from
Oran. Having shipping difficulty. Good to be back with Robertson. He

is still as funny as ever and I can laugh at his every move. Leigh and Gordon here. Guess it's true about being on Gordon's team. I'm rather pleased.

Friday, July 2, 1943

Into town this morning. Got a ride in a jeep and thought I was gonna be killed. They're calling it Hitler's secret weapon.

Half the group moving out in the a.m. for Constantine. I'm not in this bunch.

Saturday, July 3, 1943

Was told this morning that I'm to move with group this afternoon. Gordon not going yet. Destination is a place somewhere near Constantine at site of 3rd Aux.

Left Algiers at 8 p.m. aboard an ambulance train—third-class coaches and again eight to a compartment. Hot as all hell on the train and no place to stretch out. Train rides are the worst thing I've run into over here. Slow jerky trains stopping every little while so that we actually average 10 miles to the hour. And more K rations. I guess it could be worse.

A letter from Marion caught up with me—June 15. I wish I was home.

Monday, July 5, 1943

Never felt so much heat in all my life—126 in the shade—and a dry hot wind blowing continually off the desert.

Camped in a bare, open, very dry field right next to 3rd Aux three miles from El Gurrah and about 30 miles from Constantine.

Assigned to Madding's team [General Surgical Team 6: Madding, Kennedy, and Schneiderman]. We're going to a British general hospital in Tunis.

Thursday, July 8, 1943

This morning Taylor, Madding, and I had a two-hour ride in a Flying Fort [B17 Flying Fortress]—the field of the 2nd Bomber Group is right near us. We rode in *Tadilur* at about 12,000 feet. I sat in practically every seat in the ship—from the tail to the nose. It is truly the queen of the sky. Learned today I'm going to 98th British Hospital in Sousse.

Germans opened great offensive in Russia yesterday—30 armored divisions involved. Reports say fighting is terrific and casualties heavy.

Friday, July 9, 1943

This morning Gordon, Taylor, and I went over to the British tank school and learned all about our General Sherman tanks—had a good ride and even drove one for a while.

20 team captains left today for Mateur by truck. This whole move seems to be all muddled up, but then everything this organization does seem to be that way.

Loads of B17s going out every morning. 108 went today. They all seem to get back too.

Saturday, July 12, 1943

News today of Allied landings on Sicily. How the fighting is going is not told but official reports say things are going according to plan. (When I think how close I came to being there!) Went into Constantine and heard all sorts of rumors there—as always. Saw a movie and had dinner, then home by truck.

We're leaving here tomorrow at midnight by train for Mateur, some 230 miles away.

Weather quite cool now.

[The Allied invasion of Sicily (Operation Husky) began on the night of July 9–10. By August 2, British troops under Montgomery and American troops under Patton had established a line from the north coast of the island to Mt. Etna, confining the Italian and German defenders to an ever-shrinking area of the northeast. Concluding that this position was indefensible, the Axis forces initiated an evacuation on August 11 via the Straits of Messina. The Germans in particular succeeded in evacuating considerable equipment and troops by the time Montgomery and Patton met in Messina on August 17 and secured the island.]

Tuesday, July 13, 1943

Railroad thru Regada, Guelman, Souk Abras, Gnardimaou, Souk el Arba, Souk el Khemis, Beja—wrote these names down so I'd have a record of where I've been—slight change—didn't go to Beja but to Tunis instead thru Medgez al Barb. The country all along the railroad is strewn with evidence of recent war. Foxholes—burned-out tanks and guns—C ration cans—and frequently a lonesome grave. Marked at times with an iron cross topped by the soldier's helmet but more often only a crude wooden cross stood on freshly turned dirt.

Wednesday, July 14, 1943

Headquarters set up eight miles from Bizerte on what is known as Hospital Road. About six station hospitals set up and ready for work. Campsite is nice—strangely enough.

Went into Mateur this afternoon and saw demolished houses, bridges blown out, burned-out German tanks and guns—and some of ours too. Place is seething with activity right now—ammunition dumps all over the countryside.

Thursday, July 15, 1943

Got word today that we leave for Sousse tomorrow by truck. I have been running around like a chicken with its head off today—collecting men and nurses. Going to have a nice bivouac area here eventually.

Found some more German hand grenades here today—they seem to be hatching out. Bizerte has been completely leveled. Not a single house was left untouched. Our air force really did a thorough job.

Friday, July 16, 1943

A day of tarfu ["totally and royally fucked up"] traveling. Trucks showed up an hour late and without trailers. Trying to load them systematically while a few dozen well-meaning officers added suggestions was difficult, to say the least. Started our roundabout trip at 11, first to Tunis, then on to Sousse. Leigh and Havens got off at the 71st in town. Hurt is across the road from us at the 70th. Ours, the 98th General, is about five miles from town out on a dusty winding road located in and about an old olive grove. Is a 1,200-bed hospital but are running a low census. Practically no surgery at present. People seem very nice. Enjoyed seeing Tunis on the way—the docks there were almost completely destroyed. Town itself not bad—nothing like the wreck of Bizerte.

Saturday, July 17, 1943

Spent most of the morning tagging around with the chief of Surgical Service seeing the hospital. We are to take over a tent and will set up an operating theater. Have no wards to care for—nothing to do but operate. Now all we need are some patients.

Swimming this afternoon—the water here is quite warm—nice sandy beach but no surf. Dinner late—at 8—and not so good. These meals don't make me happy.

Monday, July 19, 1943

I'm afraid that this job isn't gonna produce much work—to date we've done nothing and we're getting restless. Madding is tearing his hair out for want of something to do. The entire group is fed up with the British—I was anxious to see what the group reaction would be. They have a way of making you feel so welcome—at first—and then you get the idea that it was all for a purpose. Maybe we're using ourselves as a norm too much—whether it's so or not, the British are a very different lot—and are difficult to know. There's something so much warmer—so much more real about Americans!!

Tuesday, July 20, 1943

Feast and famine—and today we had our feast. Gordon and I were on call for routine stuff and had just finished an acute appendix when we got word that a convoy of P.O.W.s was coming in. In an hour we began getting patients. All Italian and German prisoners. The wounds were the worst I've seen so far. One comminuted compound fracture of a femur looked like a cannon hit it. We ran one case right after another 'til late at night. Did three amputations, among other things. It satisfied our appetites for surgery for a while.

The Italian prisoners are in awful shape—they're emaciated and dehydrated. The Germans, on the other hand, looked good.

Wednesday, July 21, 1943

Rode an ambulance to the beach today and had an excellent swim. There was a good surf, which makes it better. Harbor at Sousse filled with ships.

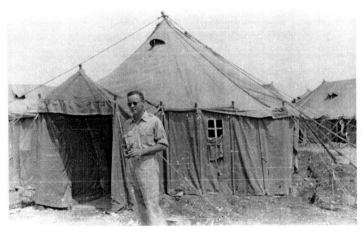

Gordon Madding in front of the operating theater at Sousse.

I'm using my free time, which is considerable, for reading and studying surgery. Madding is really a storehouse of knowledge and is good incentive to study.

There isn't a moment in the day during which I don't think of Marion—whether she's delivered or not—how she is—and what the baby is. Compared to some I guess it's not the most difficult life I'm leading, but believe me I hope it doesn't go on much longer!!

Thursday, July 22, 1943

Replastered some of our cases today—most all of them are doing fine. One of the enlisted men talks German and on quizzing the patients we find that almost all of them are sick of the name Hitler—they're tired of war. The Italians are tickled to death to be captured. One little fellow working in the O.R. has a grin on his face all the time.

Had our first death. A large soft tissue wound of the thigh died—of shock. Was in bad shape when operated—wound grossly infected and practically whole thigh shot away.

Americans almost at Palermo and 8th Army around Catania. Fall of Sicily is imminent.

Monday, July 26, 1943

The war news today was very encouraging—this morning we heard of the fall of Mussolini and this afternoon of the pope's plea to the Italian people asking them to make peace—also that martial law is the order in Italy. General opinion here is that Italy will capitulate very soon.

Tuesday, July 27, 1943

Had a few cases this morning—removed a foreign body from a chest wall— X-ray man previously put a needle on it under the fluoroscope. Made it easy.

Madding and I have had some very interesting discussions with Colonel d'Abreu,[17] chief of service. He's a 37-year-old fellow—a Catholic—and very brilliant—wrote part of Bailey's book. Gonna watch him remove an f.b. [foreign body] from a lung tomorrow.

Madding is really a storehouse of energy—he has boundless enthusiasm for surgery and all that pertains. I will learn something and will profit if I can capture some of that.

Wednesday, August 4, 1943

Up at 6:00; an ambulance took us to Sousse, and after arranging for a ride to the field we had a good breakfast—hotcakes. Just made the plane—a DC-3—as it was about to take off. Once we were in the air we learned that its ultimate destination was Sicily so we decided to tag along. At Tunis we picked up 5,000 pounds of cargo and some 30 more passengers. Flew along at 200 feet above the water—radar can't pick up the planes at that height. Landed at Gela at 12 noon. Sicily looked much like Africa but the people were actually dirtier than the Arabs. Looked in one home and saw a horse in the living room—one corner of the room was his stall. Saw Tom Ballantine [Henry T. Ballantine, general surgeon][18] and team at a medical battalion in Gela. Left Sicily at 3 p.m., and after flying a half hour we came over Pantellaria—nothing more than a large rock jutting out of the water. Back in "Tun" at 5 and in Sousse at 6. Found three letters from Marion waiting for me but no "real" news.

Thursday, August 5, 1943

Had two good cases today—a group of Italian prisoners happened along over a mined area near here and set one off. It blew them in all directions. We cut and sewed for a couple hours on our two.

Radio told of fall of Catania today—taken by the 8th Army. Germans now retreating along the coast road at foot of Mt. Etna. Orel and Belgrade have fallen to the Russians after many days of hard fighting.

Schneiderman finally got a good line on a car—a Renault which is being fixed up—painted, etc. Now we'll ride in style.

Saturday, August 7, 1943

This noon Colonel Forsee blew in. Along with him was Colonel Berry—chief of surgery in the 9th Evac. He's from Roosevelt Hospital in New York. The big news of the day is that 18 of our teams are on the alert to go somewhere with the 5th Army—and listen to this—I'm one of those alerted. No question—it's to be Italy. I don't know just what my feelings are but I'm certainly not afraid—of that I'm sure. I'll see some war first-hand 'cause frequently in landing operations the "medics" land first. Colonel brought lots of mail but no news from Marion.

Tuesday, August 10, 1943

Like the day before—that can be said too often of a typical day here in Sousse. We're quite busy with our two wards, though, and that's a real consolation. Gordon and I always manage to have four or five cases a morning. I'm doing a good bit. "Mr." Schneiderman and G. are always in argument. The only way Ben can really put anyone to sleep is to bore them to death. He's an extremely poor anesthetist and I can't say I blame

Gordon. He gives a lousy anesthetic and then always has an excuse. They had a real set-to today. Poor Ben was really laid out proper.

Saturday, August 14, 1943

Today was a very happy day for me 'cause I learned for the first time that Marion had given me a new daughter—Ruth. Chance that I saw a *Stars and Stripes* of August 7 in which I read in the lists of births about Ruthie's birth on July 23. We had a little celebration here tonight in the mess— American steaks, scotch—which I sponsored—and then a very flattering talk by Colonel d'Abreu. He is a most capable fellow and will one day be a prominent name in English surgery.

We made another trip to Al-Qayrawan and got a load of supplies so we'll be well fed for a while.

This evening Gordon and I sat outside the mess tent talking with Colonel Laird and Colonel d'Abreu. Enjoyed the evening very much.

Sunday, August 15, 1943

Said a prayer in church this morning for Marion's and Ruthie's safety. I feel much better now. Mail still is a lost item so don't know the particulars—but at least I've heard that we have a new daughter.

Took all admissions today—had one appendix, among other things. It was a tough one—Schneiderman's spinal didn't work, then he couldn't get him to sleep with ether, so the odds were against us.

Tonight we had almost a complete eclipse of the moon—all but a little sliver was blacked out.

Wednesday, August 18, 1943

Mail came in big bunches today and so now I know firsthand all about Ruthie. Fred Jarvis came down in a truck today to pick up the boys at Al-Qayrawan but they had already left. It seems there's a five-team superalert right now which we're not in on. However, our orders are supposed to be on the way. Did little of anything today except get lots of mail—some as old as May 8—all seem happy with baby. Seven pounds, six ounces and doing well.

I'm happy to know that everything is all right.

Monday, August 23, 1943

Next morning (24th)

Cleared out our wards today. Orville finally called the colonel today and he's sending transportation down for us. He said he was anxious to get Gordon and myself back so maybe we're going someplace,

Went into town—we wired the ignition of Schneiderman's car (he had gone to Tunis) and drove in. Met Captain Lewis at the officers' mess and we had a gin drink which was really potent. I had two and it went directly to my head—just a good buzz. When we got back to the hospital a couple air corps men who came to see our nurses had an alcohol fruit juice drink which they offered to us—and we took one. Now don't misunderstand, I wasn't drunk, but I did have an awful good edge on. Went over and took 120 pictures of X-rays for Hodson, the X-ray man, and now I'm afraid to develop them.

Thursday, August 26, 1943

Lyman Brewer drove in this afternoon with two trucks with instructions to return in a.m. with all aboard. Hurt's team staying with 71st, although they're not working.

Made some more last-minute hauls. Got two more quarts of scotch and more candy. Took Lyman down to the mess and got him a couple ice-cold Tom Collins, then had a good meal—went swimming bare tail off the main route of Sousse previously—this tickled him no end. His wife just had a baby boy July 27.

We've made some good friends here and I've enjoyed meeting these people—it's really an education—but I'll be glad to get back to camp.

Monday, August 30, 1943

Got three regular letters today which made me very happy—one from Marion and two from Uncle Jack with lots of pictures of the kids. Paulie and Joanie are growing like weeds but are growing nicer each day. Joanie is a beauty—how I'd like to be able to be with them and to see Ruthie, and of course my lovely Marion.

Tuesday, August 31, 1943

Orders came in today for the alerted teams, so here I go—Madding is the ranking major so will be in command. I don't know whether I like the assignment or not now that I'm on. I want to see acute surgery but I'm not at all anxious to get myself "kilt." I have too much dependent on me for that to happen.

I rode into Bizerte today and if I hadn't seen it I would never have believed it—the amount of destruction there was. Now the place is alive with activity—like the dead coming to life.

Wednesday, September 1, 1943

Orders came today—we're leaving by truck at 7 a.m. for Cape Fabeau just west of Ain-el-Turk—a three-and-a-half-day trip. There we're to join a small (400 beds) evacuation hospital. It's a real good assignment and we're more than anxious to get going. We're with the 5th Army and from what I can gather this is the big moment. As much as I have believed that Italy was the next step, I can't help thinking that we're going into France.

Mail today from Marion and Auntie. I wish I could tell them how very much I love them—Marion, darling, I love you—and with all my heart no matter what happens.

Thursday, September 2, 1943

Up at 5 a.m.—everybody flying around doing last-minute packing. I've really lightened my load this time—sold a lot of stuff and sent another box home. Swingle [Hugh F. Swingle, general surgeon][19] in charge of loading the trucks—all seven of them—he had things all snafu. Off at 8:30 a.m. to join a truck convoy of 100 trucks—we're to be in Oran by Saturday—so we have quite a ride ahead of us. Came out thru Bizerte, Mateur, Beja, Souk el Kemis, Souk el Arba, Guardimans (Tunisian-Algerian border), Souk Ahras—this latter town was the birthplace of St. Augustine.

We're bivouacked for the night in a field just outside of Souk Ahras—to be up and away at the break of dawn.

Eating K rations—we're down to bare essentials now.

Friday, September 3, 1943

We've stopped in Setif for the night—pulled in at 8:00—into a regular convoy resting post—running water and all modern conveniences. We all plunged right into a shave and a good washing which, I promise you, was a treat at this stage of the game. Had some cold cereal, tuna fish, and peaches and it tasted pretty good. Cots with mosquito nets mounted in all ways seem to blossom forth. We traveled about 220 miles today through rather barren and monotonous country. The extensive wheat fields astound you.

Have my radio with me, of course, and so tonight we heard of the landings made in southern Italy by the British and Canadians. As the announcer dramatically put it—the fortress of Europe has been invaded, and so it has. What are we headed for?—is it southern France or along the west coast of Italy—even England is mentioned in the speculation that continuously runs rampant.

Sometimes I'm amazed at the situation I'm in—lying here on a cot just about in the middle of some 100 trucks in a little town most Americans still don't know and in a country that until less than a year ago was a land of much mystery but is now colonial U.S.A.—on my way to a boat which will carry me God only knows where. I hope that all this is necessary but more than that I hope it's worthwhile.

[The landing in Salerno (Operation Avalanche) was characterized by political intrigue as well as military operations. After the fall of Sicily, Mussolini was summarily dismissed and imprisoned by King Victor Emmanuel. He was succeeded as prime minister by Marshall Pietro Badoglio, who immediately announced that Italy would maintain its alliance with Germany and just as quickly started secret talks with the Allies. Understanding that accommodation with the Allies would bring a swift reaction from Hitler, Badoglio hoped to be given sufficient time after reaching an agreement to prepare for the German response. In the event, however, the agreement they signed on September 3 was followed only five days later by Eisenhower's announcement of Italy's surrender. Germany promptly occupied Rome and subdued Italian troops in Italy, Yugoslavia, Greece, and Italian-occupied France. Hitler also sent Otto Skorzeny, an SS officer, to rescue Mussolini from his confinement. Mussolini then declared the Italian Social Republic in northern Italy.

The landings in southern Italy had been preceded by the British Eighth Army's crossing of the Straits of Messina on September 3. While the British turned north toward the invasion beaches, the Americans debarked with difficulty below Salerno on September 9. The Germans—including the troops that had escaped from Sicily—quickly counterattacked, with considerable success; indeed, they almost drove a wedge between the British and American forces. By September 12, in fact, the situation was so tenuous that the official history of the Scots Guards describes "a general feeling in the air of another Dunkirk."[20] But the crushing weight of Allied artillery, naval guns, and aerial bombing deployed against German counterattacks eventually carried the day, and by September 18, the Germans had concluded that the Allies could not be dislodged from the beachhead.

The Germans then began a fighting retreat toward the first of a series of defensive lines, the Gustav line, which ran from Gaeta on the western shore of Italy to Rescara in the east. John Keegan describes vividly how well suited the Italian terrain was for defense: "The peninsula's central mountain spine, rising in places to nearly 10,000 feet, throws numerous spurs east and west towards the Adriatic and Mediterranean. Between the spurs, rivers flow rapidly in deep valleys to the sea. Rivers, spurs and mountain spine together offer a succession of defensible lines at close intervals, made all the more difficult to breach because the spine pushes the north-south highways into the coastal strip, where the bridges that carry them are dominated by natural strongpoints on the spurs above."[21]

Moreover, in Field Marshall Albert Kesselring, Hitler deployed a strategist well able to exploit the advantages conferred upon him by the geography of Italy. Referring to his German opponents, General Sir Harold Alexander, commander of the Allied armies in Italy, said, "He is quicker than we are, quicker at regrouping his forces, quicker at thinning out a defensive front to provide troops to close gaps at decisive points . . . quicker at reaching decisions on the battlefield. By comparison, our methods are often slow and cumbersome."[22]

The result for the Allies was the long, arduous, and bloody Italian campaign, a grinding virtual stalemate that ended only when the war itself did.]

Saturday, September 4, 1943

A slow long day—this one spent in an uncovered truck beneath a blazing sun. Left Setif at 5:45 a.m. and for three hours I was frozen—gradually the sun came up and spread a warm air rather quickly. The land we traveled through was much more fertile than any I've seen—numerous orchards—peaches, figs, and pomegranates. The vineyards are being picked and the grapes harvested. The vast fields are dotted with small dump carts into which the many workers continuously pour their pickings.

Saw a mean accident—it happened right under our nose. Half the convoy was held up, so tonight we're bivouacked just outside Algiers on the road to Blida. Set up in an olive orchard along a large vineyard—the olives aren't ripe but the grapes are.

Sunday, September, 5, 1943

Still traveling and it seems we're going slower than ever. We were supposed to make Oran tonight but we stopped 80 miles short at Relizane. This is the worst place we've hit yet—just a large dusty field—not a tree or a bit of shade for miles around. And to make matters worse we have no water except for drinking. I'm beginning to realize that "this is the army."

Monday, September 6, 1943

Arrived this morning at our bivouac area some eight miles from Oran— just a rocky, hilly, barren spot called "Cactus Flats"—there's no cactus and it's not flat. Our tents are pitched on a 60-degree angle and I'm afraid I'm gonna roll out of bed any minute.

From the sound of things we're "pretty hot" and will probably clear here in four days. I guess it's Italy from all the talk here—we're attached to the 5th Army—34th Division. We're going as a group and will be assigned when we reach our destination.

Tuesday, September 7, 1943

Had a good night's rest and feel good. Hot as all hell in the daytime but cold at night.

We're attached temporarily to the 69th Station Hospital—I knew them in Casablanca.

Went into Oran with Gordon this afternoon and got all our francs changed to "invasion money"—gold seal.

We're gradually collecting equipment and by tomorrow we'll be ready to roll. Go into woolen clothes tomorrow.

No mail, of course—and won't have for weeks, I guess.

Wednesday, September 8, 1943

Big news tonight—Italy surrendered unconditionally. Italians instructed to aid Allies in every possible way.

Thursday, September 9, 1943

Learned today that we sail in a week. News of Allied landings in the Bay of Naples—contact had already been made with the Germans—feel sure we're going into Naples. The Italian Armistice was signed on September 3 but wasn't announced until yesterday, the day before the landings at Naples. There's certainly a lot of intrigue going on that precedes all these large movements and no doubt saved lots of lives.

Monday, September 13, 1943

Had a good night's rest—with the help of a little Nembutal. Went into Oran with Gordon and Hugh Swingle this morning. Swingle is a character—a nice-looking fellow from whom the words flow like water. We went to the docks at Mers el Kebir and saw the *Durban Castle*, the boat on which we're to sail. It's a large boat—is English. Drove out to Ain-el-Turk with some instructions for our nurses. Ate dinner at a mess in a villa high up overlooking the sea—a beautiful place—and had an excellent meal.

Tuesday, September 14, 1943

Word today that we load in a.m., probably will sail the day after. Spent the morning getting my stuff lined up. Went into town this afternoon—took my cot with me that I broke this morning. I was fortunate enough to get a brand-new one—they're scarce here and will be an impossible item in Italy. Had a shower at the Officers' Club (without a towel), then a sandwich—and back to "Cactus Flats" for our last night. We just beat the rain home—it came down in buckets and just about washed us off the hill. First rain since last spring and it's making up for lost time. Had a regular river running under my cot all night.

Wednesday, September 15, 1943

Up at 6 for early Mass—bright moon shining. By the time we finished breakfast it was again raining cats and dogs—water poured right through the tents and we were quite thoroughly soaked. By truck to Mers el Kebir at 11 a.m. Fortunately we were able to get our trucks fairly near the boat so we had only a short carry—finally boarded at 3 p.m. I'm rooming with Weiss [William A. Weiss, Schneiderman's replacement as anesthetist][23] on A deck—have a fairly nice room—much better than that on the *Elena*. First meal was very good—nice piece of beefsteak—but as always they're short of water. We pulled out of Mers el Kebir at 6 a.m. and sailed into the Port of Oran—a distance of three miles—for the night. Rumor says we'll be here for a day or two. Radio reports of fighting in Italy are poor.

2

Southern Italy and Monte Cassino

Thursday, September 16, 1943

Water is turned on at 6:30 so Weiss bounces out, washes, fills all canteens, helmets, and draws a basin of water for me—before it's turned off again at 7:00 a.m. We're still in Oran—little bit of loading going on all day and now we're all set to go. Rumor has it that we'll sail sometime during the night. Saw minesweepers go out this evening, which suggested that we're about to move. Little of anything to do—nice officers' lounge but of course is very crowded. Played bridge most of this afternoon—think I'm improving. Radio reports much improved and suggest that tide is turning. Story goes that original plans called for easy occupation of area around and south of Naples.

Friday, September 17, 1943

Up at 6:30 for Mass—disappointed to find that we were still tied up at the Key. Tony Emmi giving a few Italian lessons—had a two-hour session with him this afternoon. Boat pulled out into harbor around noon—rest of convoy making up around us. Bridge for several hours this afternoon with Weiss, Madding, and Miss Hussell—I'll never be a bridge player. We pulled anchor at 6:45 this evening. We're the flagship and so we're riding the center of the convoy. Sea is quite calm and there's practically no roll to the boat.

Radio reports contact between 8th and 5th armies. 5th now on offensive. Good!!

Saturday, September 18, 1943

Mass at 7 this morning—there's a good attendance.

Only nine ships in our convoy, escorted by six destroyers—we're running along the African coast about 10 miles out. An occasional Spitfire flies over us. A troopship alongside of us is flying a barrage balloon. Making about 12 knots an hour. Sea very calm. Supposedly passed Algiers at 2 p.m.

Playing bridge much of the time but I still am not an expert.

Sunday, September 19, 1943

Dawn found us still running along the coast—general consensus of rumor says we're opposite Tabarqa. Weather still perfect but sea is a little more rough. Passed an island at 7 p.m. Jahlita, which lies just off Bizerte. Debarkation orders put us fifth in line—not decided yet whether we'll land at a dock or beach.

Just watched a convoy of 30 ships pass us—came awfully close—had their running lights on and we did ours. Hope we weren't too conspicuous. We were concerned about a brilliant flaming light hidden by clouds way off to our port side—turned out to be the moon.

Monday, September 20, 1943

Still all is uneventful—weather perfect and sea calm. Sicily has been on our starboard side all day. Passed many small islands which jut up out of the sea like huge rocks. Large formation (72) "Forts" passed over us this noon. Told this afternoon that we're debarking early in a.m. by means of small beach craft. Guess is it will be on beaches below Salerno although the Port of Salerno is in our hands.

I'm anxious to land in Italy 'cause I'm looking forward to working again and also I'm eager to see the sights it offers. No country in the world is more steeped in history. This is a great opportunity but I'd chuck it all to be back with Marion and the kids.

Tuesday, September 21, 1943

Up at 4:15 a.m. for an early debarking but as always with the army we hurried to wait. Dawn revealed Italy, mountainous and rugged, just a few miles off our starboard side. We were approaching the Salerno beaches from the south. By 8:00 we were among numerous ships of all makes and types—L.S.T.s [landing ship tank] L.C.I.s [landing craft infantry], freighters, destroyers, cruisers, battleships, and many transports. Debarked at 4:15 p.m. by means of L.C.I. boats onto beaches. Could hear heavy artillery rumbling in the hills constantly—that plus the yellow warning flag (air raid imminent) suggested the possibility of trouble. We immediately started out for 34 Division headquarters in a truck. After riding 15 miles in the direction of the front we were sent back to the exact place we had left. Pitch dark, cold, damp, and everybody hungry. Gave up at 9:00 and just laid down on the ground for a bad night.

Wednesday, September 22, 1943

Of all the miserable nights I have ever spent last night was the worst. Just 100 yards off the beach, no blankets, nothing but a towel to wrap up in. I shivered practically all night and got about 10 minutes' sleep. Gordon out early to 5th Army headquarters—came back with the news we're all attached to 8th Evac. Found out all their equipment had been sunk so they in turn are attached to 16th Evac. Half of our teams that landed on D-day are with 16th. They had an exciting time and as they say were scared to death. The landing was known in every detail by the Germans—they even had maneuvers here three weeks previous to the landing. Russell's group from Sicily brought in here on D6 with 45th Division. They're with 93rd Evac but aren't working.

Colonels of 8th and 16th had words this afternoon and the 8th moved out across the road—mad—so we're with them. (The war is going on in spite of all this). I have my bed set up and I'm all set for a good one.

Thursday, September 23, 1943

I'm used to anything now—I couldn't sleep on the *Durban Castle* but in the open it's a different matter. Our pup tents are up—look awful but are more comfortable. Many of group that came from Sicily were over today—all have transportation and so will probably get the first assignments. Meant to mention the mountain stream that runs behind the hospital—it's fed by springs and the temperature is below 50—but oh, how refreshing it is after this heat. Temperature here has been around 100 but like Africa the nights are cold and two blankets are necessary. Do our washing and bathing down in the stream.

Friday, September 24, 1943

Still sitting in our pup tents behind the 8th Evac. I will say that their meals are 100% better now than when we were with them last. Some of the Sicily groups have been assigned to the small evacs, including the 94th, so I guess those are out for us for the present. Can still hear the guns at night and see flashes over the hill. Early this morning Jerry bombers were over the harbor (beach) and dropped a few bombs but did no damage.

Got orders this afternoon that we're being attached to the 16th Evac again—just across the road. I'm afraid they're going to resent our coming, however. Nurses of the 16th Evac came in tonight. They were torpedoed on the way over.

Saturday, September 25, 1943

Salerno—just two and one-half miles behind the enemy lines ahead of our own artillery and under the range of Jerry. Got assigned to civilian casualty hospital at noon today and arrived here at 5 p.m. tonight. As we approached Salerno we drove right thru the middle of an artillery barrage—ours. The loudest and most startling thing I've ever heard. We're attached to a British A.D.S. [advanced dressing station] and probably are the most advanced American medical unit. The point to which ambulances go is only one mile from here. Salerno is on the sea, closely crowded in by steep hills, beyond which our friends are settled. Right now shells are flying over us—and to say the least, it's disconcerting. Not set up to work as yet but will be tomorrow.

Sunday, September 26, 1943

A busy day trying to get our operating room all set to go. We're under AMGOT [American military government for occupied territories] and they're working on a shoestring, I believe. We're all set now and will start operating in a.m. All day long we were besieged with patients—civilian casualties—but of course we had to refuse them admission. Artillery firing over our heads all day and I'm quite used to it now. Last night they fired continuously and I didn't sleep a wink. The hills in back of (east) Salerno go right up straight and attacking up them was difficult—getting the casualties down is even worse. Tonight they say Jerry is pulling out. No shells dropped in town all day so I guess we're safe. Moved to better quarters today.

Monday, September 27, 1943

This place seems to be just one headache after another—trying to get sterilizers, autoclaves, etc. in Salerno is a difficult problem to solve. We're open for business and did a few minor cases. Sort of a general practice in Salerno. Went through the other civilian hospital today, from which many of our cases are coming. I never saw anything like it—up numerous flights of cold stone tunnel stairways through big, drab, and bare foul-smelling wards, flies all over every patient, practically covering every stinking dressing—these people are a backward lot. A bomb was exploded near here today. Artillery still firing over our heads but much less.

Tuesday, September 28, 1943

I really never knew the definition of the word *madhouse* until today—from early morning until late tonight we were going constantly—just one case after another, and the sad part of it is that they're mostly children. One little kid about five years old lost both legs and an eye—had five amputations altogether—did three eye enucleations and two of them were on kids. We've got practically nothing to work with and there's so much work to do. Food is a real problem—how they're going to eat is beyond me. AMGOT is an organization that has little more than a headquarters, yet it expects wonders. I never really knew until today what war means to civilians—it isn't just rationing, doing without, and all that, it actually means pain and suffering and death in many cases. I feel thankful to God that mine are safe.

Wednesday, September 29, 1943

Dawn to dusk—that's one day and every minute of it is full. We do one case after another but at the end of the day we always find more new cases than we did that day. Supplies are still a problem but we're doing a little better. The post-operative and nursing care is still practically nil, so the outcome of many of our cases is many times very questionable. We have about 82 patients now but only enough food for 10 and only for another day—just one of a million problems. That little kid we cut the legs off yesterday died today—better that he did.

No mail from Marion plus this discouraging work puts me right in the dumps.

Heard today that Naples was in ruins—much cholera and typhus there—is off limits already to all troops.

Thursday, September 30, 1943

The days fly by here and are really getting shorter. Lots of work makes time "fugit." Have done 36 cases, mostly majors, in last three days. Got a new civilian doctor today, that's a real help. He does all the ward work and it's changing all the chaos to something that is gradually resembling a hospital. Had a case of full-blown tetanus come in today—first real one I've seen. We had a variety of cases that makes the military hospitals look sick—all good stuff. Gordon says we'd better just stay here and open a clinic in Salerno. There is no question about it, medicine and surgery are on a low reach here in Italy—same in North Africa too.

Friday, October 1, 1943

Heard today that in the recent storm the 16th Evac tents all blew over and that there was real chaos for a while—they had some 1,200 patients. Our quarters are perfect now—single rooms, cleaned every day by one of our Eyetie [British slang for "Italian"] ladies. A hard floor and four straight walls are hard to beat. Hope this lasts for a while longer.

Saturday, October 2, 1943

Busy from morning 'til night with much work still ahead of us. We have asked so many people for supplies that finally we're getting a fair supply. Weiss and Gordon got into it hot and heavy today—one thing led to another until finally G. told W. that he didn't know a damn thing about anesthesia. G. is so cocksure of everything. I found out, much to my surprise, that few in the group like him. He has been very fair to me.

Sunday, October 3, 1943

Called out of early Mass to do a suprapubic cystostomy—fellow hadn't urinated in three days. Again had our hands full. Did a Callandar's amputation, my first of that kind. I'm getting to do a lot of things that I've never done before. Had one fresh compound fracture of leg.

Took a walk down into town at noon—first time I've been out of this place since we landed. Salerno was deserted then but now the people are back in large numbers. It was a pretty town once but now is in ruins. Quite a few ships in the harbor. Looks like they are going to use the port since Naples is out. Had another case of tetanus develop—boy age 14—in five days—phosphorous burns.

Monday, October 4, 1943

Work much slower but we're still busy—have a chance now to give more post-op care, which is important. Major Sullivan [James M. Sullivan (eventually lieutenant colonel), commander of the Second Auxiliary teams supporting the 7th Army] up today and brought our equipment. He went on to Hurt and Wolff [Luther H. Wolff, general surgeon],[1] who are in rear of 45th and 3rd Divisions. Brought a little mail but none for me. We're living in fine style now—even running water in our rooms— that came on today. These "Eyeties" really appreciate us and do everything they possibly can for us. Gordon going to supply area tomorrow for food.

Tuesday, October 5, 1943

Things were too good to be true—this morning shortly after Gordon had left for Paestum (for supplies) we got orders to go immediately to the 8th C.C. [casualty clearing station] in Naples. Just when we were really working. Had about five very interesting cases come in, which we turned over to the 14th C.C. to do (had one arteriovenous aneurysm). Gordon was sick when he came back with the loot. Left Salerno at 5 p.m. in a British lorry loaded to the ceiling. First real sight I've seen in Italy loomed up shortly before us—Mt. Vesuvius—belching a large column of black smoke. The road wound around it and as evening came you could see flames leap from its center. The mountain itself is surprisingly small. Drove into Naples in pitch darkness. Couldn't find the C.C.S. so we're sleeping tonight in a corridor of the postal telegraph building—a really modern and beautiful place.

Wednesday, October 6, 1943

Up at 6:30—had breakfast with an A.P.O. [army post office] outfit. Drove around Naples a little and saw a little bit of it—it's been hit very badly but the place seems heavily populated. The Germans were here only five days ago and certainly left a trail of destruction in their wake. The last thing they did was to blow up the complete power plant. The water system too was destroyed. Finally found the 8th C.C.S. about five miles out of town in what was once a contagious hospital. Very nice outfit. Had met most of them at Sousse. One other surgical team, so believe we're in for quite a bit of work. Line now is 20 miles north of here at the Volturno River.

We're starting the 4 p.m. to 8. a.m. shift—not good but it's for two weeks only. My darn bursitis is back again and it hurts.

Thursday, October 7, 1943

Started this afternoon at 4—we're on from 4 p.m. to 8 a.m., which is a rather long and tiring pull. Cases here are on an average of 10 hours old. Had a good head case and an amputation of a lower leg. Amputations don't interest me very much—I've had too many of them. The way they work it here, you just stand in the operating room and they bring the cases into you. The system works pretty well but you neither see the patient before or after operation. All preparation and post-op care is taken care of by general duty officers. Our capacity is 350 beds and tonight we have 550 patients, so there's no more room. Otherwise I wouldn't be getting to bed at 1 a.m. (Better mention here that as I look out my window now I can see Vesuvius glowing in the distance.)

Friday, October 8, 1943

Nothing came in after 1 a.m. so got a pretty good night's rest. Hitched a ride into town this morning—found the fellow was going near Pompeii so we rode along with him and walked all through the ancient ruins (a few modern ruins were mixed in with them). The preservation is quite remarkable and some of the mosaic is just as if it was laid yesterday. Some paintings in an old house of prostitution were also remarkably preserved (they would be). Vesuvius first erupted in 63 A.D. and then again in 79 A.D. The last eruption was in 1926.

Not admitting tonight—house still full. Did five cases this evening so we're all cleaned up.

Saturday, October 9, 1943

Had an air raid in the early hours of the morning but it wasn't much. Yesterday a delayed mine exploded in the building (the new postal building) in which we slept our first night in Naples and killed 100 people—just two nights previous I had an uneventful sleep there.

Not busy here—there's a C.C.S. ahead of us so I don't imagine we'll get much real work. Feeling is we'll move very soon. The line is about eight miles past the Volturno now at a line of hills—the last defense before Rome. When that falls they'll be to Rome in no time.

Raining constantly for past few days.

Tuesday, October 12, 1943

Business is still slow but a terrific barrage has been going on about 20 miles up the road. We were off tomorrow and had planned going out near Pompeii to buy some cameos but we've been instructed to stay close to home in case a big push is starting. The unit was alerted earlier in the day—we're supposed to be moving up but if things have started already we may stay here.

Monday, October 18, 1943

Up at 6 and away by 9:30, which is pretty good considering the size of the unit. Took us about an hour to go in convoy (30 trucks) the distance of 18 miles from Naples to Santa Maria. The roads of course are cluttered up with pretty heavy traffic going in both directions. We're located in an Italian school right in the center of town—place is a little crowded but we have a good-sized theater—at noon we were all set to go. There's a F.D.S. [field dressing station] across the street with an F.S.U. [field service unit] attached so they're taking 30, then we take 50 cases, so we're closed until they get 30. This seems like a pleasant town—not much physical evidence of war. There's plenty of noise, however—we're right in line with the heavy artillery and they're blasting away full blast all the time. We're just three miles from the Volturno at and across which the fighting is taking place.

Wednesday, October 20, 1943

Didn't get to bed until 5 this morning so I'm sleepy right now. Cases coming in heavily but we've got three teams working now, which is a help. I'm seeing and doing more stuff now than I ever hoped to—it's good, of course, 'cause it makes the time fly. Some of these boys are pretty well shot up—one fellow today had a piece of shell in his brain, a bullet in his belly, and his left hand blown off. All the cases are like that—not one injury but a dozen. They come in here exhausted—tired and filthy dirty. Some haven't been out of their clothes in weeks. I think the more lightly wounded are pleased sometimes just to get away from it.

Thursday, October 21, 1943

Little to do last night so in bed by 12. Had one interesting case—an American with a "stove-in" chest. The recoil of a large gun caught him and practically every rib was broken. His chest wall just fluttered in and out with every respiration.

Had an air raid at 7 this evening that lasted over an hour—no bombs dropped near here, but someplace—likely Naples—took a pasting.

Saturday, October 23, 1943

Big influx of patients—started working at 4 and finished just now, 2:30 a.m. One officer patient had a terrific wound—almost all his bladder was shot away—nice-looking young major. Four letters today but only one from Marion.

Sunday, October 24, 1943

Worked until 2:30 this a.m.—had a real busy night and saw some good stuff. One major's bladder was blown to pieces—Gordon did a nice job on it. Did a tracheostomy for the first time. Slept until 11 a.m.—getting used to this night shift now and rather like it. Went next door to 12:00

Mass this morning and again there's a different routine about standing and sitting—no kneeling at all.

Cases have stopped coming in so we're playing a little bridge tonight. There's a case in now—don't know what it is but must leave to do it.

Monday, October 25, 1943

This is my last day on the graveyard shift. This noon we drove over to Maddaloni, about eight miles from here, to where the 94th Evac is set up. Saw all our group and we were able to scrounge a few things. They had just received several strafing cases which were hit just a mile out of Santa Maria. Two Spitfires (manned by Germans) came sweeping down on them. They supposedly have some Flying Forts, too.

Tuesday, October 26, 1943

We started our new hours at 8 this morning—it's midnight now and we're quitting only because our time on duty is up. We've been busy every minute of the day. A sucking wound of the chest that I sewed up this morning died this evening. That's our first death here.

Major Price (the F.S.U. team) is back in the hospital so we're getting a new unit tomorrow—also we're supposed to be moving again. Don't know where 'cause we can't go much forward or we'll be ahead of the artillery again.

Wednesday, October 27, 1943

Started right in at 8 this morning and worked 'til 3:30. Most all of our teams are being sent out—presumably to field hospitals. Stopped in at the 8th Evac at Caserta on the way back. Saw Robby and got a letter from him (from Marion). Back here to find a load of cases, so we pitched in and worked until 11. Made chicken sandwiches and coffee afterward—tasted pretty good. Then to finish the day I took a hot bath (in a canvas bathtub two feet by two feet).

Thursday, October 28, 1943

The 21st C.C.S. moved in and so is taking patients every other eight hrs. Somehow we always happen to be on while we're receiving and consequently are very busy. Things are running more smoothly now and seem to be getting even better.

Jarvis came in for tea—his team is temporarily with the 8th Evac at Caserta. The 15th and 16th Evacs are over there too—that puts four large evacs right together. The front in that region is almost 30 miles up but here it's just 10. We can still hear the artillery even though it's almost two weeks since we arrived here. Cases are taking a little longer to reach us, however, about 10 hours—which still isn't too bad.

Friday, October 29, 1943

The F.S.U. attached at present (Major Escort and Captain Kennedy) along with Captain Pitpaine have been ordered forward. Four F.S.U.s are being sent across the river about eight miles. Supposedly a big battle is about to start. Major Burge and team also leaving. We'll be shorthanded and consequently swamped here. Went over to Caserta to medical supply—located in the summer palace of the king—a spacious and beautiful place. Back here to find Madding and Weiss up to their ears in work. Had several big cases.

Jarvis and a couple other teams assigned and leaving today for clearing stations. Every one of us is now busy.

Saturday, October 30, 1943

Not admitting from 8 to 4 p.m. so we took a little walk around the town. Found out that this was the original Capua—now called Santa Maria Capua Vetere. It was here that all the gladiatorial fights took place—this was the locale of Spartacus. We climbed all thru the amphitheater where the shows were held—saw the dens where they kept the lions—might even have walked into the room where Spartacus charged the gladiators. Hitched a ride over to Capua—it's in ruins—saw the Volturno—fighting 10 miles from there.

Admissions starting coming in at 4 p.m. and we were swamped. Did 28 cases—worked 'til breakfast and here I am Sunday morning ready for bed. The battle is on but not 20 miles away.

Sunday, October 31, 1943

Up at 4 this afternoon after a weird night. That 4 in the afternoon to 8 in the morning shift is a killer. Had one sucking chest wound die on us; that's the second one we lost. They appear to be minor wounds but actually they're very major. We did 28 cases during the night—that's the most we've ever done at one sitting. Again I say I've had my fill of this war surgery—all I want to do now is keep moving, seeing the country, always getting closer to home—so far I haven't headed that way. Also at this point I'm again a little tired of the British. There's plenty of good work here but you have to talk an awful lot before you get it.

Monday, November 1, 1943

Meant to mention that the other night while we were prepping a patient on the table he rolled over on his side and as he did two nice grenades dropped off on the floor—makes it a little worse when you realize he was a Jerry. Had five cases up 'til 12:00. 21st C.C.S. admits from 12 to 8 so although we're on we'll sleep all night (a year ago today I left Kilmer and home).

Wednesday, November 3, 1943

That poor mail distribution must have upset me terrifically 'cause here I am in the 38th Evac Hospital. I've had diarrhea for some time now but during the night I really got sick—headache, cramps, and fever—so this morning we decided to go for mail so I could get sick in an American hospital. This hospital is a good one located near Caserta. I have a fever and my head still aches, but I don't think I'm very sick.

Had a V-mail dated October 8 from Marion today—she hadn't heard from me in two weeks. I guess that covers the period I spent coming to Italy.

I sorta feel guilty being in this ward—mostly all surgical—legs and arms gone, etc.—my diarrhea looks a little cheap.

Thursday, November 4, 1943

Feel much better today—had a good night's sleep with the help of a little Nembutal. Stomach better and my guts have just about quit—temperature normal too so I'll get out in a.m.

Gordon and Weiss in this afternoon with news that we're moving up the road about 20 miles. Mason [James M. Mason III, general surgeon] and his team are coming with us along with four other American nurses—we'll have Miss Stratton [Lina J. Stratton, nurse][2] too. Back to tents is the only sad part of it.

Friday, November 5, 1943

Completely well and so I'm leaving here as soon as I can get a hot shower (a real luxury)—had it and it was delicious. Bummed back by way of the castle and stopped at the A.P.O. Much to my great surprise I got about 12 letters and a lot of it from Marion—had my first look at Ruthie—a snap by Uncle Jack—she's very pretty and I do believe she looks like me. Also a picture of Paulie and he looked awfully sick in it. One of Joanie too— she's a beauty. Lots of interesting stuff in Marion's letters—they're really wonderful and help no end.

Miss Stratton is with us once again. Don't know if that's a help or not.

Have to be up at dawn ready to move. Air raid tonight—not much.

Saturday, November 6, 1943

Slow in getting away and we're held up for two hours trying to cross the Volturno at Capua. Jerry ruined that place and as usual blew all the bridges.

One-way traffic over a pontoon affair slows things up—very pretty country—quite hilly—lots of signs of war plus artillery booming in the distance constantly suggest this isn't Pennsylvania. We're set up in a farm (no buildings) just outside of Sparanise. We're reduced to a tent again but our pyramidal isn't bad—we have a stove in it which is a dandy.

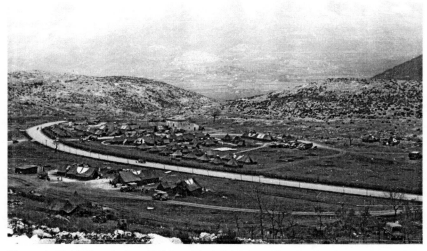

Eleventh Field Hospital and Thirty-Sixth Division Clearing Station at Sparanise.

Sunday, November 7, 1943

Froze half the night though I was covered by everything except a gun. Started a fire (Weiss did, rather) in our stove early this morning and it heats the tent beautifully. Went to Mass at 7 a.m. in this little farmhouse next door. If we're here next Sunday I must get a picture of it. Have an F.D.S. next door and they admitted today so we were off.

Heavy artillery fire going on most of day—at night it lights the sky brilliantly. Ack-ack firing all around but I saw no planes.

Monday, November 8, 1943

Got a rush of patients in so we had to work last night—got in bed at 3 a.m. Had one good case—a transverse wound of the liver. Busy all day today—mostly little stuff except a bladder and gut perforation. Place is still a sea of mud but sun out all day. My Arctics are coming in good—from Danville to Italy.

Heard Hitler on the radio tonight—shouting all over the place saying that the Russians have now been stopped and that they (the Germans) are ready to go on the offensive in Italy—where does that leave us?

Always a group in to hear the news—quite a picture—Madding in the corner taking a bath—half a dozen over the stove and the beds loaded—the radio and the stove make us very popular.

Wednesday, November 10, 1943

Had a very unpleasant air raid early this a.m. I was very suddenly awakened by a terrific noise and associated shaking of the cot—a bomb dropped about a mile from here—lasted for an hour or so.

Little work today—they say there are a number of casualties up in the hills near the Garigliano River which they can't get to. New F.S.U. arrived today—8th Army outfit—that leaves us free to be called out of here, which we think will be soon. Progress has been nil the last few days—the Garigliano is still the line—yesterday the Jerries made nine counterattacks down this main road to Capua but without much success—lots of noise, however. Here we are 10–15 miles from the war but all one hears of it comes from London.

Thursday, November 11, 1943

Up and out of here by 9 a.m.—we're off until 8 tonight. Hitched a ride up to the 94th Evac. They're five miles northeast of us on the main—everybody working there right now. The 3rd Platoon of the 35th Field Hospital (Larry Hurst [CO of the platoon]) are eight or nine miles ahead of them. This morning at dawn they were heavily shelled (not bombed) and had to evacuate the place, leaving all belongings behind. One officer killed (not ours). One shell fragment drove into the sterile table, another hit the oxygen tank against which Paul Hutchins [Paul F. Hutchins, anesthetist, later assistant orthopedic surgeon and assistant general surgeon][3] was leaning as he was giving an anesthetic—close.

Friday, November 12, 1943

Little work just before noon. Went up to 94 in search of the 33rd Field

1st Platoon. Got a ride on up about 10 miles and found them located just ahead of the artillery—what an awful noise—funny, in a few minutes you can get used to it. They're quite busy—Wolff's, Shefts's and now Sully's [Sullivan's] team—doing only A1 priority cases. Stopped back at the 94th for dinner—they had steak and I ate three—first meat I've had in Italy.

Saturday, November 13, 1943

Another new schedule today; we're on 12 hours and other team on night 12, then off tomorrow—all piddling stuff coming in for which there's very little to do. Heavy artillery barrage started at 2 a.m. and lasted practically all day. There's one particular hill on the top of which is a monastery under which are many passageways. Jerry is entrenched there and they're just about leveling the hill to get him out. It's interesting to try and piece the stories together—what you learn is much more like the truth than what the B.B.C. news gives out. They've attributed the hold up here to bad weather—the sun's been shining for past 10 days without a break.

Monday, November 15, 1943

On tonight at 8 so we've had little or nothing to do all day. Raining continually and this place is a sea of mud—reminds me of the *Big Parade* or *All Quiet on the Western Front*—as I remember them. There's been no progress up ahead. The artillery has been thumping away from the one spot for days—night and day. I guess those prisoners weren't so far off when they said they were going to hold the river for eight weeks. With the weather the way it is, I think we'll be sitting here for a long while.

A tent in the rain and mud all over everything and the end of all this seeming so far away—Christmas coming on—it just isn't a happy situation.

Wednesday, November 17, 1943

After the rain the mud sticks around—and everything sticks in the mud. That's the way it was here today—everybody a foot deep in it. At least we had heat—we were able to trade the farmer here for some wood— gave him tobacco and bully beef. I think he got the worst of the deal. No work at all.

They say both Americans and British on this front had to give a little ground. Jerry dive-bombed a bridge a few miles up the road and knocked it out. That really slows up things.

Friday, November 19, 1943

The sun came out and stayed out all day—that's a record. My gut's on the blink again and I'm sure it's nothing but the damn food. I'm eating so little of it now I'll be thin as a rail before we get out of here. Colonel told us this afternoon that we have now been released by X Corps, which means orders will be here for us any day. A new F.S.U. came in here to take our place.

Today's my birthday—31 years. I used to think that was an awfully old age but I don't think so now. It seems only yesterday that I was just a kid—and now I have three of my own. I hope this is my last birthday away from home.

Saturday, November 20, 1943

More rain—wonder where that phrase "sunny Italy" ever started. Gordon and Bill went into Caserta—borrowed Major Jack's truck. I stayed home 'cause my guts were still saying no. Got our orders today to go to II Corps. We think it means the 11th Field so we're happy. Truck coming Monday to pick us up.

Had Jerry planes over several times today—low-hanging clouds give them plenty of cover. They dive-bombed a bridge twice about a mile from here (didn't hit it). One plane was hit—smoke just billowed from it and then it took a nosedive. Roads near here were strafed too. A shell went thru the cab of one of the C.C.S.'s trucks—fortunately it didn't hit the driver. Mail today—five from Marion with some good pictures. We bought the drinks in the mess tonight for group—farewell party and had a good evening.

Sunday, November 21, 1943

Last Mass in the farmhouse—tomorrow we move. Still raining. Weiss incapacitated by last night's party but will live I'm sure.

A few planes over here this afternoon but did no strafing. Yesterday 6 out of 11 were shot down. They actually strafed the main street of Santa Maria where we lived a few weeks ago.

Monday, November 22, 1943

Awoke to find the sun shining—how much easier that makes moving. Our British pals seem sincerely sorry in having us leave. Packed and ready by 10. Adjutant from 11th Field (the place we hoped we'd make) came shortly and informed us that a truck and ambulance would arrive at 1. 11th Field set up behind us near Capua. 3rd Platoon is at "front" with Wolff, Adams, and Sullivan. We're to go out tomorrow with 1st Platoon. Looks like good assignment. Good chow (fresh roast beef tonight), hot shower, and lights in our tents. We're even burning soft coal. These Americans know how to go to war. Incidentally, we're set up in the middle of an orange grove.

Tuesday, November 23, 1943

1st Platoon moved out today but we're not moving until tomorrow. We're going to be behind the 3rd Division and at the moment they're not in the line. We'll be bivouacked about five miles behind the front. The 3rd Platoon had its kitchen hit by an 88 last night—a nurse and two enlisted men were wounded. They have the darn thing set up right in among the artillery (Long Toms), so what more can they expect? More rain here today and there's mud everywhere.

Wednesday, November 24, 1943

Up early to find the sun shining but by the time we were ready to strike the tent it was pouring—a five-minute wait brought the sun out again. Moved up to 1st Platoon—set up at junction of Capua-Roma and Riardo road. We're serving as a surgical hospital for the 3rd Division while they're in rest. Then when they go into combat again we'll follow them doing only priorities (good setup). This is a good area—nice O.R., etc. Major Boylen in charge with two other M.D.s.

Thursday, November 25, 1943

Thanksgiving Day—had a real turkey dinner with all the trimmings and it was the most delicious meal I've had in a whole year. This outfit knows how to live.

George Donaghy and a couple others were here for dinner—they're up four miles with our 3rd Platoon and are being shelled day and night. They have their cots sunk down in foxholes six feet deep in their tents. They are sitting right in the middle of field artillery, and ours and Jerry's shells and noise are driving them slowly crazy.

Raining all day and a real downpour most of the time—the mud is getting deeper.

Friday, November 26, 1943

A very remarkable day—the sun was out all day—first time in weeks.

Threw a football a little bit (my bursitis is still with me, I find). Had a couple cases, minor things.

Rather a big air raid on tonight—lasted for an hour or so. Flares on parachutes made the place look like day. Believe they were aiming at the palace in Caserta. Gives you an awfully unsafe feeling not to have some kind of a roof over your head.

Sunday, November 28, 1943

Did a couple minor things and then went to Mass down at the clearing station of the 3rd Division. Hitched over to the 94th this afternoon and rode up to the 3rd Platoon of this field hospital. They're about six miles ahead of us. They've had a tough time—one shell knocked their kitchen out and others have fallen near them. They have their cots sunk down inside foxholes. The guns all around them start at dark and continue shooting long into the night. They frequently hear a German shell whistle over their heads and they say that it seems that each one is coming in the tent with them. There's a hill a few miles ahead on top of which a few Jerries stay lodged. As we watched it, B24s came over (12) and bombed it.

Monday, November 29, 1943

Just doing some plain unadulterated sitting right now but heard this morning that we're to move in a week. The 3rd Division is all set to go into the line up the next valley and we're to follow them.

The last half hour the big guns have been booming away constantly. It's surprising how used to it you can get—that's at a five-mile distance, but right in among them it's a different story. It will always remain a mystery to me how soldiers in the line can face the things they do. No one will ever know just what it's like, but I think we come the closest to knowing.

Thursday, December 2, 1943

Tonight there's a barrage going on and I'm sure if it keeps up much longer they'll knock over the mountain they're trying to take. It's just about continuous and sounds more like machine guns rather than artillery fire. The sky is lit up just like it used to be when they had fireworks at Rocky Glenn, only—much worse.

Tuesday, December 7, 1943

Drove into headquarters of the 11th Field this morning after breakfast to pick up some more instruments. Went on over to Caserta to the A.P.O.

but found no mail—very little for anybody. Back at noon. Colonel up here today inspecting—fortunately the O.R. looked very good.

The Italians supposedly are taking over a small part of the front and they have a concentration right next door to us—what a motley-looking crew they are—last night I heard one of the enlisted men say, as he was helping to get an Eyetie truck out of the mud—"My God, but I'll bet the Germans are laughing at us now."

Thursday, December 9, 1943

Days are long and mostly very empty—time to be passed. Whether or not anything happens, the excitement or interest of it is merely a scratch on the surface of my great loneliness. The only saving factor is the knowledge that sometime it will end. How I could ever face a permanent loss I do not know.

Had a 20-year-old good-looking young redhead brought in tonight—shot thru the abdomen accidentally. He died before we could do anything for him. A telegram for somebody just in time for Christmas—"We regret to inform you—."

Friday, December 10, 1943

Just another day for most people, but for one Ina Mae in Iowa it's just about the end of the world. She doesn't know it yet but she will—over in the 41st F.A. [Field Artillery] Battalion they had accident—practice firing the rocket gun—one blew up. Killed the captain and injured five others. We got them all here hours later—too late to do anything for Corporal Warren—an arm and a leg blown off plus a thousand other wounds—he died. So tonight, unknown to her, Ina Mae Warren is without her husband—and forever. Just one little story that is being repeated every hour of each day and as long as this war goes on.

Monday, December 13, 1943

There seems to be a lot of activity going on around here—boats going up the main road. They say that the Germans are moving stuff for a heavy counterattack—an armored division fellow told me that this afternoon. It seems that every time we get ready to do something the Germans anticipate it and counterattack first. There has been practically no movement for days now. I think Italy is fast becoming a headache to the Allies.

Tuesday, December 14, 1943

Heard today that we move Friday the 18th but to where we don't know.

There is still a little talk about an amphibious movement but I sincerely hope not. Weather is clearing—roads a little drier so maybe we are going soon.

Got Dad's Christmas card today and really enjoyed it. Paulie, Joanie, and Ruthie were beautiful and I felt really proud of them. Sometimes my loneliness really adds up to an actual ache that I can feel and that hurts—and the end seems so far away.

Friday, December 17, 1943

Finally got some mail today—G. [Gordon Madding] went into headquarters. Four letters from Marion, which were good—I can almost hear Marion saying what she writes in her letters. Sometimes I don't think I'll last—I'll bust or just go nuts longing and wishing for her.

Endless parade of bombers over today with large fighter escort. Hardly ever see an enemy plane and Hitler's latest is that he rules the sky over Italy.

Saturday, December 18, 1943

The 3rd Division is on the move—more stuff going by here than you can shake a stick at. The medical battalion is moving and the rumor has it that we move Monday.

Bombers still parading north over us in endless procession. It's only a short while until we hear them returning.

Read an article in an old *Jersey City Journey* this morning. Headlines—"Rail Junction of Averra Taken by Allies." Sounded important—actually the town was a burg—one small single track running through it. Baloney for home consumption.

Sunday, December 19, 1943

Four weeks have passed since we joined this outfit and still we haven't moved—but it's in the offing. There's more stuff going by our door than you ever could imagine. To Mass again at the clearing station. They won't be there Xmas so if we're here, we'll have to find a Mass. Got an Xmas package from Mom and Dad H. today—won't open it 'til Christmas.

Monday, December 20, 1943

No word about moving as yet. Hospital practically empty and nothing coming in. Walked down by clearing station through the woods looking for a Christmas tree. None to be had. Clearing station all packed and ready. There's a natural spring down there, but the bottling works are all blown to hell. There are numerous natural springs or spas in Italy. The regular drinking water is very poor. I went to a movie tonight over at the 94th Evac—in the pouring rain. Saw Chester Morris in *Wrecking Crew*, a real dog—a crime to ever send a picture like that over here.

Friday, December 24, 1943

Christmas Eve—and though it's far from what it should be it's much better than last year's—and I'm much closer to home. The nurses put on a cocktail party at 4. Had the tables all nicely decorated—candles and poinsettias—they all had evening dresses on and looked very nice. In the evening at 7 they put on a party for the men. Had wine and fruitcake—sang Xmas carols too. Went to midnight Mass at the 15th Evac down the road. Had an organ and a fiddle with a choir. Very Christmassy, but so very far from home.

Saturday, December 25, 1943

Christmas Day—my second one overseas and my last, I hope. This was a little more pleasant than last year—people here made a little more effort. Maybe too it's 'cause we can't help but feel that the war can't last too much longer (but if we don't move any faster than we're moving in Italy, we'll be at it for years). Had a delicious turkey dinner with all the trimmings. The nurses had the table set with candles and poinsettias and it was pretty. I ate 'til I thought I'd bust—had to take a nap afterwards. Raining again—at home it would be snow. I couldn't help but feel awfully lonely today. I miss Marion more each day, it seems.

Tuesday, December 28, 1943

Just got all set for a few days at Capri and we suddenly get alerted. We're moving about 12 miles from here and only a few miles behind the front. Hospital is half apart already.

Bill Nelson sent over eight turkeys and so tonight we had another real dinner. Had Cliff James, Macfarland, and Pitpaine over to enjoy it. They ate like starved pigs. Had alcohol and fruit juice afterward in our tent (Yocky-Dockies). Wind blowing and it's cold as the devil.

Wednesday, December 29, 1943

Moving tomorrow morning, so we'll be getting war casualties again. Went over to the 38th Evac this afternoon and spent the afternoon and evening there with Bill Bowers drinking Spanish cognac. I had a little glow but nothing radical—had roast beef. Reeve Betts there plus a few other teams. Invited back for New Year's Eve but don't think I'll be able to make it.

Thursday, December 30, 1943

Up at 6:30 and packing for a 12-mile move. Moved into new area on Route 6 few miles short of Mignano. We had been in the area for an hour or so—everybody unloading and putting up tents, etc., when suddenly there was a terrific explosion about 20 yards from where we were standing—dirt, parts of a truck, rocks, and general debris started falling all around us. The truck had been driven over a land mine. Engineers were called in and four mines were found. One was just outside our tent door where everyone would walk over it. Takes 200 pounds to set one off.

Friday, December 31, 1943

It's 9:30 p.m. and I'm about to go to bed—not that I'm tired, it's just that there's nothing else to do—and sleep lets you dream. It's been raining cats and dogs all day and our area is almost completely underwater. The tents are leaking, making everything miserable—makes you wish a thousand impossible things—and you end up by feeling awfully sorry for yourself. Only bright spot of the day—went to Mass at 6 p.m. And so 1943 ends. Great advances were made—that can't be denied, but it's hard to apply them locally (I'm still thousands of miles away from home—and Marion). Here's a prayer and hope that in 1944, with the war won, I'll be home.

Saturday, January 1, 1944

Back at headquarters for a brief period, and of necessity. A terrific storm blew up just as the new year came in and laid the hospital low. A 90-mile-an-hour wind, rain, and snow knocked all the tents down and spread equipment all over the area. I got soaked through several times and by dawn we had to give up. Evacuated all our patients and took off for headquarters. I don't think I ever spent a more miserable night and hope never to have another like it. Going back in the morning to try and collect our stuff.

Sunday, January 2, 1944

Still at headquarters but we had word tonight that we're to be back at the 11th Field first thing in the morning, set up by noon. Will be glad to get away from this place, but it certainly was nice to have someplace to go when we were rained out.

All kinds of rumors circulating—we're going to England—there's another invasion, etc.

Monday, January 3, 1944

Back with Unit I, 11th Field Hospital. Got here at noon and found place fairly well set up and just about ready to function. Still just a quagmire but our tent stood up all through the storm and so it was fairly dry inside. Got a little mail today—one from Mom (H.) telling me lots about Ruthie, Joanie, and Paulie, and I feel awfully lonesome right now—if I could just see my family for a day—just see them and hold them in my arms, I'd feel better—but no, damn it, I can't.

Just finished a patient—bad fractures of both legs and blast injury of chest—pretty bad.

Tuesday, January 4, 1944

Shells fell during the night and uncomfortably close—I thought we were supposed to be out of artillery range. Our case of blast and fractures died this noon—he was a Britisher. When I was closing out his record I happened to glance thru a prayer book that was his and noticed a little verse that he had underlined. The markings looked years old but what I read was very appropriate—something from St. John: "—whosoever believeth in him should not perish but have life everlasting." I hope he has it.

Three more teams joined us this evening. Word is there's to be a big push tonight.

Wednesday, January 5, 1944

This is really early tomorrow morning but I'm just going to bed so I'm writing a little late. Very early this morning—2:30, I think it was—I was awakened by the scream of artillery shells racing over our heads. Never really heard them so clear and distinctly before, but there was no question as to what they were. I don't know what Jerry was firing at but it seemed that we were his target. We've been awfully busy the past 24 hours and every case is a real emergency. One fellow came in with his brain half out—another had the entire half of his jaw shot away. We've had to remove half the bowel in some cases. There's an awful lot of good work here. It's cold in the O.R.—so cold that early this morning ice formed on the sterile drapes. The patients are all in shock when we see them and it's a job to get them fit for the O.R. The ward tents are cold and the wind blows through them like a bat out of hell. Most of these patients would be touch and go even under ideal conditions, so what chance have they here? It's very obvious to us here that the war is still far from won. We can't even take Cassino, let alone Berlin. Much more of this winter in Italy and I'll have had more than I want.

[The Monte Cassino massif provided the Germans with a nearly impregnable site for the western anchor of the Gustav line. In addition to its formidable defenses, it commanded Highway 6, the principal western route to Rome. The capture of the mountaintop was therefore critical to the advance on the Italian capital.

So strong was the German position that three attempts to take it between February 12 and March 23 were repulsed, despite heavy aerial bombardments that reduced the Benedictine monastery atop the mountain to a jumble of ruins. It wasn't until mid-May that the Polish II Corps finally succeeded in dislodging the defenders, opening the way to Rome and sending the Germans into retreat.

General Mark Clark, commander of Fifth Army, then faced a strategic choice: drive northward across the rear of the retreating German Tenth Army to try to encircle and capture it, or take Rome. Ever conscious of his image and reputation, Clark chose the role of triumphant liberator of the Eternal City and let the Tenth Army escape.

Clark's vainglorious decision allowed German field marshal Kesselring to conduct a fighting withdrawal, completed in August, to the Gothic Line, running from Pisa in the west to Rimini in the east. He was to hold this line virtually until the end of the war, prolonging the bitter stalemate on the Italian peninsula.]

Thursday, January 6, 1944

Slept through breakfast, didn't get in bed until 4 this morning, and a full night's session it was. I'll be an old man in no time flat if this keeps up. It was so cold early this morning in the O.R. that ice actually formed on the inside of the tent.

Friday, January 7, 1944

Off at 4 p.m. tonight, but we had just started a case which took us till 7. I'm dead tired and ready for bed. We've been working without a stop since 12:00 last night and we've had some pretty big cases. Some of the wounds and injuries we're seeing are amazing. I'm really sick of war surgery—it's awfully depressing to see young healthy boys shot up like these.

Colonel Forsee here this evening—there's another invasion and some of our teams have to go. Gordon gave him a flat no and a very emphatic one when he asked if we were interested. I hope we don't make the team.

Saturday, January 8, 1944

Working most of the day but cases not coming in as fast as they were. Didn't get much sleep last night 'cause Jerry shells were falling short of us—sounded as if they were in the tent with us. I tried to sleep with my helmet over my head but it wasn't very successful.

Heard from the colonel tonight that our team isn't on this next job. I feel more relieved than I can say—'cause I don't wanna get "kilt" at this late date.

Learned today that in eight or nine days there's to be another big push up ahead of us—also we're going to move soon.

Tuesday, January 11, 1944

The short lull was broken today—a shell just landed and not very damn far away—I don't like it!—had a couple pretty bad cases in but we're getting rid of some so things aren't too confused at present. The 3rd Platoon is going to leapfrog us and we're going with them. Will be six miles up this road and it's too close for me. The teams going on the invasion left by boat this morning.

Wednesday, January 12, 1944

A slow day—no new cases. We're gradually evacuating the hospital and now have only 10 cases left. So far we've only lost three cases but there's another one that's a little touchy. Weather continues to be like a late spring day—about without a jacket most of the day—a week ago we were freezing. 36th Division going by us all day. Advanced party of Major Bonham's platoon (3rd) going up ahead of us tomorrow. Question as to what's to happen to us at this point.

Thursday, January 13, 1944

Didn't sleep worth a nickel last night—shells were falling just ahead of us and a few sailed over our heads—in the dead of night lying on a cot in a tent it seems like you're in the most exposed place in the world—but they never seem to quite reach us exactly.

Did an amputation on a British boy today—he was heartbroken when he found out he had to have his leg off.

Friday, January 14, 1944

I've come to another stagnant period in my diary. Radio gives great praise to the French attacking Cassino from the east and northeast. They supposedly are all set for a big push against Cassino but so far there has been nothing doing. We still have shells landing on our doorstep and if you stop to think about it much it's a very uncomfortable feeling. Weather now is perfect—warm days and cold nights.

Sunday, January 16, 1944

Up at 4 a.m. this morning to do a belly case—fellow had a large hole in his colon and a comp. comm. [compound comminuted] fracture of right femur. Finished just in time for breakfast. Mass at the clearing station at 10 a.m. There's still doubt as to whether the other platoon is going. The Germans are pulling out of Cassino and the report is that the road beyond it to Rome is crowded with German vehicles. Took a walk over the hills today—beautiful country right now. Back to a good turkey dinner. Movie tonight—Orson Welles. Sounds like a day in the States.

Monday, January 17, 1944

Business picked up again—the 141st Infantry of the 36th Division has been advancing through areas filled with booby traps and we have been getting the traumatic amputations—had five come in today—I did one.[4]

Wind is blowing up and the temperature is dropping—I'm afraid we're in for some more winter. Our artillery is now five miles ahead of us and they're blasting away continually almost all day long. Haven't had anything come this way in several days now—which is good.

Four letters from home today but none from Marion—and that's not good.

Tuesday, January 18, 1944

Major Bonham's platoon is finally going to set up—about five miles from Cassino near a town that was taken only five days ago. We'll be about five miles ahead of our own artillery. Seems to me we'll be right in the middle of things. O.R. busy all day—we're on the graveyard shift tonight—midnight to 8—here's hoping we get by without getting up.

Friday, January 21, 1944

Got word this morning that we were needed at Major Bonham's platoon so we struck our tents and left Major Boylen after lunch. Rather sorry to leave that group—they were awfully nice to us. Good chance of being with them again, however. We're really in the war now—some of it is actually behind us—our own artillery. Fortunately we're set up between two hills which gives us some cover, though not much. We're beyond Mignano almost near San Pietro.

Colonel Ginn [L. Holmes Ginn Jr., II Corps surgeon] here—said landing was to come off early tomorrow morning below Rome in an effort to cut off General Kesselring. Did two cases tonight—to bed at 1 a.m.

Saturday, January 22, 1944

It's really tomorrow—2 a.m.—but I'm just getting to bed for today. Early this morning—about 4 a.m.—we were awakened by the scream of artillery shells flying over us and then by their explosion, some of which actually reached our cots. We could hear the German gunfire, then hear the scream and with our breaths held could hear them explode. It went on until 7:00. I promise you I was scared to death. We've been busy all day—some tremendous wounds. New landing made below Rome, successful and unopposed. Our forces driven back across the Rapido River again. They've crossed it twice now. The place is alive with mines.

[The "new landing made below Rome" was Operation Shingle, which was launched in an effort to insert a force behind the Gustav line and threaten Rome from the west. The U.S. VI Corps achieved complete surprise and landed unopposed at Anzio, only thirty miles south of Rome. Rather than attempt to exploit the surprise immediately and push inland, however, the American commander, General John P. Lucas, contented himself with landing men and equipment and solidifying his position. The Germans moved so decisively and effectively to counter the landing that when Lucas did attempt to advance toward Rome on January 30, he discovered that he was surrounded and trapped against the sea. The Americans and British then found themselves confined to a small beachhead. Initial German attempts to attack and annihilate the beachhead were repulsed with difficulty and with heavy losses on both sides. Thereafter, Allied forces were subject to almost constant aerial bombing and artillery attack. Lucas was relieved on February 23 and replaced by General Lucian Truscott, to whom fell the duty of holding the beachhead until Cassino finally fell to the Allies on May 17, thus unseating the western anchor of the Gustav line. Finally, on May 23, VI Corps broke out of Anzio and joined the push toward Rome.

History has perhaps been kinder to Lucas than his contemporary superiors. In retrospect, it appears that his mission was, at best, ill defined. Rick Atkinson goes so far as to call his orders "muddled and contradictory."[5] Lucas has been faulted for not lunging at Rome upon landing, but it is not clear that he had the resources to do so successfully. Keegan says, "Had Lucas risked rushing at Rome the first day, his spearhead would probably have arrived, though they would have soon been crushed."[6] Indeed, Gerhard Weinberg places the blame for the failure to exploit the success of the landing squarely on the shoulders of Clark himself: "Incompetent leadership by General Mark Clark . . . allowed the opportunity created by the initial surprise to pass unutilized."[7]]

Sunday, January 23, 1944

Went to 10:30 a.m. Mass over at the 111th Clearing Station—Father Murphy, a Franciscan. General absolution and to Communion.

Only a few casualties coming through. A Brigadier General Kendall [probably Paul Wilkins Kendall, commander of the Eighty-Fourth Infantry Division] went thru this morning. Said we were forced back over the river. Supposedly the Germans asked for a three-hour truce this afternoon for time to pick up the wounded and to bury the dead—it was refused.

There's a lot of artillery banging away right now. German shells are going over us, breaking in the valley to our rear. Can even hear German machine guns—not good, McGee.

Monday, January 24, 1944

Rooted out of bed at 3 a.m. for a case and didn't finish 'til breakfast. Got in bed and wasn't disturbed 'til after dinner. Fellow had bilateral comp. comm. femur plus large and small bowel wounds. Heard this afternoon that we lost 700 men on the other side of the Rapido. We've been pushed back completely now but there have been no attempts at crossing by the Germans. Shells fell just over the hill during the night but none within a half mile of us. We're only four and a half miles now from the river— uncomfortably close. Radio reports good progress by the troops just landed. We're hoping they draw Jerry out of here.

Tuesday, January 25, 1944

How do they expect me to sleep? The artillery banged away all around us all night—some new British guns moved in behind and when they fire they shake all Italy. Heard today that Johnny Adams and an enlisted man were lost when the hospital ship on which they were stationed was torpedoed and sunk off Anzio. Ruth Hindman,[8] one of our nurses, was in the "hold" ward with Johnny dressing a patient. He sent her up as soon as it happened and he stayed with the patients—and is still with them. He's the first casualty in the 2nd Aux.

There was a three-hour truce on the river line this afternoon—Germans brought 100 dead up to the barbed wire—they even rowed a few wounded across the river—then in three hours the war went on.

Wednesday, January 26, 1944

Another one of those days when it's really the next day—on first call at midnight and we worked until 7. I did a right colon.

Saw an A36 shot down up the valley ahead of us. Particularly heavy ack-ack by the Germans, then this one plane (out of 24) fell down like a dead leaf.

Very little shelling by our guns and practically none by Jerry. A fellow over in the clearing station, a litter bearer, told me the 36th Division was putting up barbed wire on their side of the Rapido. Guess they must be expecting counteroffensives.

Thursday, January 27, 1944

Got up at 10 but felt like more sleep. Rode down to Major Boylen's platoon and had lunch. They're all packed and ready to go whenever there's room enough to move them ahead of us. Heard further stories about the bombing of the hospital ship—Johnny went down with the ship. He helped Ruth Hindman get on her life belt and then he went to his ward to get patients out. Before he could get out the ship went down in four minutes. The other two hospital ships underwent nine bombing runs but weren't sunk—they were all well marked and fully lighted.

Friday, January 28, 1944

Marion's birthday—every time something happens now it's the second time it's happened since I've been overseas. I hope there are no third such anniversaries.

Did a couple cases today. One fellow, a machine gunner, had just set up his gun in an emplacement 300 yards from the Rapido, and an 88 landed in the hole with him. Large chest wound plus a complete severance of his cord—19 years old and now is just a vegetable.

Germans dammed the lower Rapido and flooded the plains in front of Cassino. Last night the 142nd Infantry Regiment was moved up to St. Elmo past Cassino in the night so tonight there may be something doing.

Sunday, January 30, 1944

Had a very active night as far as Jerry shells were concerned—from 1:30 until 3:30 they whistled over us and a few broke on the hill alongside of us. A new 240-mm gun moved in a mile behind us and has been firing all day—it sounds like it's just behind your tent. Dug a foxhole in one corner of the tent just to have someplace to hide when Jerry starts trying to find that gun. This war is getting "serial," so Adkins [Trogler F. Adkins, assistant general surgeon, later general surgeon][9] says.

Monday, January 31, 1944

Got thru the night without a case—good. Did dressings this morning—all my cases doing well. Went out in the Jeep this afternoon and saw a little of this area. Went over to Mignano—took pictures. It's the most bombed place I've ever seen. Took a picture of an American tank near there that hit a mine (900 pounds T.N.T.). Saw that 240-mm gun that's behind us. It's tremendous—fires a 360-pound shell 16 miles. Drove up beyond the hospital over to San Pietro—it's in ruins. Could see San Vittore ahead down the valley. Mt. Trocchio too and the Jerry hills beyond. The road we drove over was shelled a half hour before. Tried to get some descriptive pictures of what a war land really looks like.

Tuesday, February 1, 1944

Been awfully noisy around here all day—those two big guns have been firing over our heads constantly. Heard today that they were going to try and take Cassino tonight. Tanks have been going up all afternoon. It's hard to figure out just what the tanks are doing—one minute they're going up—the next, they're all coming back. Their area is just a mile or two behind us here.

Wednesday, February 2, 1944

Most everybody got a load of mail today—and I got one letter from Marion—my mail situation is a heartbreaker. I'm really sick and tired of all this now. I "wanta" go home!

Few patients coming in—one fellow told me they really had the Germans in a bad way—had them surrounded practically but one thing he couldn't understand—how the Jerries were firing at them from three sides.

Thursday, February 3, 1944

Took a walk up Lungo this afternoon—that's the hill alongside of us. It doesn't look very high or formidable but a climb to the top gives you a different idea. It's just covered with rocks and now it's littered with shrapnel and German and Italian hand grenades.

Halfway up the hill a Jerry 88 is dug in and well placed. It covered the road coming up the valley.

The entire side of the hill and particularly the top are covered with pillboxes. They're all well made and only a direct hit would drive you

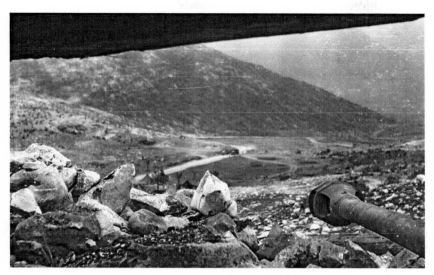

German 88 commanding Route 6, the road to Rome.

out. The hill stands right at the head of Mignano Valley and together with Rotunda commanded all that spreads before it. You can see the Rapido from there too—could see our guns firing constantly.

Friday, February 4, 1944

The rains are back with us once again. Been raining all day and this area has just about reached its saturation point. As per usual the pitch is just opposite to what we figured. Had a thrill along about 6 p.m. Jerry shells after days of silence started flying over our heads, landing not awfully far from us. The low clouds perhaps made them seem close but I am certain I could have reached up and caught one. Weiss and I had started a foxhole days before but didn't finish it. Finished or not, we dove into it and by some miracle got our heads below the ground. Tents that were foxhole-less suddenly sprouted dirt piles outside their doors and so most of us are again approaching the "mole" stage.

Saturday, February 5, 1944

And the rains went—the sun is out again—good thing 'cause this area wasn't made for drainage. Our foxhole filled up during the night so we'll have to call the war off for a while.

They're fighting now in the streets of Cassino and I guess from all reports the fighting is pretty bitter. The progress has been awfully slow—

it seems they're trying to do this particular job on a shoestring and not much more.

Still no mail from Marion. I'm beginning to wonder if something has happened to her. This is no good being over here.

Sunday, February 6, 1944

Had a really remarkable demonstration of ack-ack this afternoon. Three Me 109s flew over up ahead of us and our guns started at them. The sky was alive with black puffs and bursting shells. The pattern followed the planes wherever they went and finally one went down in flames. Several ack-ack shells fell in our area and exploded but no one was hurt. Two weeks ago there were German guns where ours are now—that's some evidence of movement.

General absolution again this morning and to Communion.

Monday, February 7, 1944

One of those "really tomorrows" (4 a.m. on the 8th). We went on at 4 p.m. and caught a load of work. Three Spitfires dive-bombed some of our artillery positions near Cassino and we got a few that were really shot up. Supposedly the Spitfires were flown by Jerries—they've done that before. Radio news from the beachhead isn't so good—some sources are calling it another Salerno. It hasn't seemed to have had the desired effect on this front 'cause the Germans are still bringing in fresh troops. The 36th is almost shot to pieces at this point.

[In late January, attempting to bypass the Gustav line and force his way onto Highway 6, the direct route to Rome, General Clark ordered the Thirty-Sixth Division to attack across the Rapido in the teeth of heavy German resistance. The results should have been predictable. Indeed, after the war, Field Marshal Kesselring said, "From a military standpoint, it was an impossible thing to attempt." At the end of three days of futile attempts to fight their way across the river, one thousand soldiers of the Thirty-Sixth were dead. "By any reckoning," wrote Rick Atkinson, "two U.S. infantry regiments had been gutted in one of the worst drubbings of the war; the losses were comparable to those suffered six months later at Omaha Beach, except that that storied assault succeeded. 'I had 184 men,' a company commander in the 143rd Infantry said. 'Forty-eight hours later I had 17. If that's not mass murder, I don't know what is.'"[10]]

Tuesday, February 8, 1944

I really saw the war firsthand today. Luther, Charlie, and I climbed to the highest and topmost and forwardmost point on Mt. Lungo. We had a full view of the entire valley in which this little corner of the war now goes on. Portia with Trocchio behind it was just three miles ahead. Behind them loomed Mt. Cairo and just over Trocchio the abbey of the Benedictine monks could be seen. Shells were bursting all around it. We could see the German gun positions far off to the left—they'd fire and the shells could be seen landing near the monastery. Screaming meemies and airbursts were plentiful. Jerry artillery had one of our gun batteries zeroed and he was frapping its A. The Liri and Rapido rivers were up ahead to our left. San Angelo on the Rapido was being shelled. Both the rail bed highway and Route 6 were alive with traffic but we could see the end of the line.

The whole valley was dotted with shell holes—there seemed to be thousands of them. San Vittore and San Pietro lined the valley to the left and thru glasses proved to be mere shells of what they once were. It was hard to believe that here right before our eyes was a real war.

On the way across the top of Mt. Lungo we came across several dead Jerries. One with no head; the other didn't seem to have a wound. I took the helmet of one. Supposedly tonight they're going across the Rapido.

Radio at noon—told of 23 deaths in an evac hospital at the beachhead. 12 of them were nurses. The radio said they were dive-bombed.

Thursday, February 10, 1944

Brewer's and Hoffman's teams left us today to join the other platoon. We immediately became very busy here—that's usually the way. Been raining here all day and is quite miserable. We were only on second call but we worked continuously from morning 'til night. There's been absolutely no progress here and even less, I guess, at the beachhead. The guns haven't moved an inch since we've been here and we're hearing just as many Jerry shells and guns as ever. Colonel [Jarrett M.] Huddleston, VI Corps surgeon [and director of medical services at Anzio], was killed at Nettuno today. Not good—too many doctors and nurses being killed.

Friday, February 11, 1944

Working quite hard and we're shorthanded. 142nd and 143rd Infantries are to do something but nobody knows what. Talked with a fellow just back from Mt. Cairo area—he told me that there's an American tank graveyard there with lots of our best in it. They're taking a beating. Jerry has tank turrets mounted on pillboxes up around the monastery. Why we don't bomb hell out of that building is a mystery to me. Little news of the beachhead but from the way everyone talks it's not going well.

Saturday, February 12, 1944

What a night—another real shelling from 3 until dawn and this time shells landed yards from us—the remainder roared over our heads like boxcars and the shell exploded as if it was in our tent. We hit the floor of the tent and hugged it closely 'til it was over. We've been rushed all day and the cases are terrific. The news is still all bad. Just a slaughter here. 33rd Field at Anzio was shelled and one of our nurses was killed, Tex Farquhar[11]—several others injured. This 2nd Aux looks like a jinxed outfit.

Sunday, February 13, 1944

My sleep is at best only fitful. I have one ear to the northwest constantly—which isn't good. It seems there's to be no discrimination as far as the Red Cross is concerned.

Our bilateral thoracotomy and laparotomy of yesterday is doing quite nicely—if he lives it will be a major victory—he was an ambulance driver, incidentally, and was driving his vehicle when hit.

Getting quite cold here but the weather is clear. Casualties slowing down. News from here and the beachhead is still poor.

Monday, February 14, 1944

Rather definite now that the 36th and 34th Divisions are coming out of the line. This field hospital is going to the rear to act as a station hospital for them so I guess we'll be out of a job for a while. There's lot of talk that we're going to England but nobody knows. Business is very quiet right now but our cases of a few days ago keep us pretty busy.

Heard today that Tony Emmi and Phil Giddings [Wooster P. Giddings, assistant general surgeon, later general surgeon][12] were wounded when the shells hit the 33rd Field.

Tuesday, February 15, 1944

Got thru the night without a case but I didn't sleep. I must confess I haven't slept well since that last batch of shells went over. Cases coming in today mostly are field artillery. They say that if they stay long enough they always get it eventually.

Talked with a Father Fenton of the 141st Regiment this morning and learned some startling figures. For every nine men they should have in the line they now only have one. One company has three men left in it. Fortunately they're all being pulled out and in three days will be out entirely.

The monastery was finally bombed by us. Several hundred Forts flew over here today and they say it's now level—it's about time.

Wednesday, February 16, 1944

Learned that Giddings was quite seriously wounded—Emmi not so badly. Supposedly somebody has to go to relieve them.

Been a lot of shelling going on all day—German shells were landing the other side of the hill from us about a mile away. They knocked out a gun and so we had several cases—all frapped up.

Thursday, February 17, 1944

Sullivan's team taken early this morning—they joined three other teams to go to the beachhead. We were told by Major Bonham that our team is gonna stay with them while they act as a station hospital—that means peace and quiet for a while.

There's more activity here tonight than we've had in a long while. There's a push on to take Cassino—started at 9:30. All New Zealanders so we won't be very busy. A 1st Armored officer told us tonight that it was a big push that just had to be successful.

Friday, February 18, 1944

Story is that Cassino fell today along with monastery hill behind it but nobody is quite sure of it. 47th Armored moved in across the road and we're gonna take their casualties so I guess we'll be here for a while yet.

Had dinner this noon across the road at medical supply—fresh roast beef and very good. Our food is lousy—plus no coal for our tents and it's very cold.

Had a movie here today—first one I've seen in months and I enjoyed it very much.

Saturday, February 19, 1944

Business as usual—just enough to keep our wards full. Got down to our friend at the Q.M. [quartermaster] today and for a quart of alcohol we got enough stuff to last for months—can of coffee and canned turkey, etc. It makes this business of living in tents a little easier.

Reports from Anzio are poor and I guess they're really in tough straits. General Martin [Brigadier General Joseph I. Martin, Fifth Army surgeon and medical planner for Anzio] was here today and said the hospitals were swamped. They couldn't get men either in or out. 93rd, 56th, and 15th Evacs there now with the 33rd Field. 50% of our teams are there.

Sunday, February 20, 1944

Still cold as the devil and no coal. Just finished a partial gastric resection—also did a splenectomy and colostomy to boot—my first of that nature.

Mass over at the clearing station and Communion this a.m.

Lost the railroad station last night in Cassino and the abbey ruins again. There's been practically no progress here and from all reports they're being just about pushed into the sea at Anzio. I'm thanking my lucky stars I didn't make that trip. Some mail from home but none from Marion.

Monday, February 21, 1944

Our gastric resection died today but it wasn't unexpected. Four more teams left for the beachhead today, and according to Luther Wolff, who was at headquarters today, it won't be long before we're all there. Some little shake-up in the outfit—nurses being transferred out—a chief nurse is pregnant—a couple of majors leaving because they refused to go to the beachhead. Seems like the 2nd Aux is slightly upset.

Had another bad night here; if shells screaming over can make a night bad. None landed near us, however.

Tuesday, February 22, 1944

A little diversion here this afternoon—had a movie but you could neither see it nor hear it so I guess it doesn't count. Had another near catastrophe at Anzio—a shell landed between Major Hopkins's and Flood's [Clyde E. Flood, assistant general surgeon][13] tents and demolished them both—fortunately all hands were in the O.R. at the time. The fighting has died down there and according to B.B.C. the Germans are being held. The hospitals are 36 hours behind in their surgery.

Sunday, February 27, 1944

One last day at this stand. Hospital closed tonight and tomorrow our teams are going back to join the headquarters of 11th Field. Luther staying here as a holding company—only two patients left. Our last one died this morning. The last three cases we did died. We came here January 21, just 36 days ago, and the front has changed very little since. Progress has been practically nil and it has cost. Two divisions are mere skeletons. Now we go back to rest while they re-form, and then where to?

Monday, February 28, 1944

Packed and left the area at San Pietro at 1100 hours after a very noisy night—shells fell awfully close last night. Got over here—11th Field headquarters—at noon. We're about seven or eight miles west of Piedmonte.

Just what we're to do here is a mystery to us and I'm afraid it won't last. Very nicely set up here—hot showers, pretty good food, and no noise.

Wednesday, March 2, 1944

Called into headquarters this morning bright and early. It sounded like Anzio for sure, but our fears were poorly founded. We were assigned to a platoon of the 10th Field that's setting up on the coast road #7, the famous Appian Way. Wolff, Swingle, Ballantine, and us. Went into Naples this evening to the Allied Officers' Club—quite a swanky club in its day. Had dinner there and then left for headquarters for the night. I almost wrecked the weapons carrier on the way home—didn't have a drink either. Starting out in the morning for Carano, where we're to set up behind the 88th Division.

Friday, March 3, 1944

Left headquarters after breakfast and arrived at Carano at noon—in the pouring rain. The 10th Field was in a muddle and seemed all confused. They have the hospital set up not at all like it should be and are not very willing to take suggestions. If you ever want to get discouraged, try pitching a tent someday in real deep mud in pouring rain. We're with the 313th Medical Battalion of the 88th Division and supposedly we'll

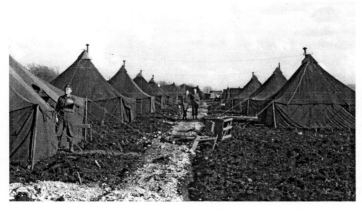

In the mud at Carano.

be busy very shortly. It's a long haul to the nearest evac so we'll be doing more than usual.

No guns behind us, thank God. Heard Gene Haverty [Eugene F. Haverty, evacuation officer, Office of the Surgeon, Fifth Army] was killed at Anzio last week.

Saturday, March 4, 1944

Still raining and now the mud is like glue. No business as yet—story is that we won't be very busy before the 9th, but we're ready now.

We're only a few miles from the coast here—today and all last night the navy parked a few miles out and continuously lobbed shells over our heads—they make a terrific swish. No guns behind us, however.

Heard tonight that the 36th and 34th Divisions have moved to Maddaloni and the 11th Field with them—to a staging area. Also, the 94th is packing for a sea trip. What next?

Monday, March 6, 1944

Business is still slow and will be until the 9th. That's when the 88th is supposed to go in. The story is that they're going to attempt to take the coast road and join up with the beachhead.

It's been a pretty good drying day—that plus many feet of duckboards makes this place quite livable. Our meals have been surprisingly good—pork chops this evening.

We're still without lights so the radios are all silent and thus no news available.

Thursday, March 9, 1944

We got a case in at 7 a.m. this morning and we were busy from that time until dinner tonight. The war must be in progress again. Our man of this morning died just a little while ago—a machine-gun slug went in his left buttock and came out his right chest. Luther got a generator from headquarters so we'll have lights. (He sent orchids to Marion, too, for me.)

More artillery banging away tonight than you can shake a stick at. This was the day set for the beginning of a new offensive—we'll see what develops. Another big daylight raid on Berlin by Forts today.

Friday, March 10, 1944

A very peaceful day—no work, so I guess nothing happened last night.

The artillery is really firing tonight and the discouraging part of it is some of it is behind us. They're gonna start that again. We could hear bombs falling—thought it was Cassino but Charlie Rife was over here today and said it wasn't Cassino. You can see Cassino area from the 94th. The 94th is packing—they think for a water trip.

Had a Coca-Cola today—first one I've had in over 16 months and it tasted pretty good.

Saturday, March 11, 1944

My patient P. went out today. Our streak of losses is now up to five. I think we've been jinxed.

[Luther Wolff noted, "The boys want to hang a sign on the morgue tent here: 'Surgery G.S. #6.' Gordon Madding's team is known as Surgical Team Number Six, and he surely has had tough luck with his patients lately. I ordered the boys not to put up the sign."[14]]

Monday, March 13, 1944

One of sunny Italy's few sunny days—quite warm. No business but there may be some before breakfast 'cause the sky to the northwest is bright with artillery flashes and the noise is terrific. Heard this afternoon from some of the boys who were at headquarters that we're gonna be pulled back to go to Anzio or someplace by water. However, the 11th Evac just pulled in in back of us five miles down the road.

Tuesday, March 14, 1944

A big day in Bill Weiss's life—orders came through on him today taking him to the States—on rotation. Here he is going from here to a place just 18 miles from home—how I'd like to be doing the same— but for me it will probably be another year or close to it. We plugged for George Donaghy to come up and be our anesthetist. No work now—things still very quiet but the colonel says we'll be busy in a week or so.

Wednesday, March 15, 1944

The long-awaited bombing of Cassino finally took place today. All morning long Forts, B-24s, and B-26s flew over us in large groups. The noise was terrific and even shook the ground at this distance. B.B.C. tonight said 14,000 tons had been dropped—3,000 sorties flown. Naples was raided last night—103 planes were over it.

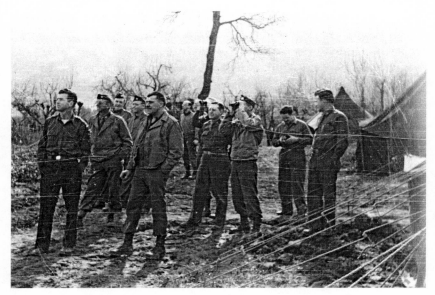

Second Aux officers watch the bombing of Monte Cassino, March 15, 1944.

Thursday, March 16, 1944

Talked with an artillery officer from the 36th Division. The tanks are a mile past Cassino and are going up the Cairo valley to the Adolf Hitler line. Still fighting at the abbey.

Few casualties coming in but very slowly. Started tearing the hospital down to put it up in the form of a cross.

Friday, March 17, 1944

Weiss left here this afternoon to begin his journey to the U.S. and Wilkes-Barre. Just thinking about it makes me more lonesome than ever. Kaplan [Irwin Kaplan, anesthetist][15] from the 80th Station took his place.

In spite of the heavy bombing Cassino still isn't all ours. The damn Jerries are being stubborn about this thing.

Still no work here—no signs of it either.

Tuesday, March 21, 1944

The first day of spring and it's raining like the devil. A tent in a muddy field in Italy can be a miserable place in which to live. Got another tent mate today—a Captain Todd Towery [Beverly T. Towery, shock team][16] from Tennessee. He's here to replace Berlin [Erwin S. Berlin, shock team, later assistant general surgeon] in shock—seems to be a nice fellow. Four in a tent plus all our junk makes the tent quite crowded.

No business—very quiet but lots of artillery these last few nights.

Radio news about Cassino is bad. I'll bet the N.Z.s will have to pull out of there.

More mail from Marion today—two regulars. Mail is a real help.

Wednesday, March 22, 1944

Business picked up a little tonight. Got three cases in and from them we drew a belly—my case. Closed two holes in the stomach. Kaplan had the devil's own time keeping the patient on the table. Maybe Willy [Weiss] for all his talk and peculiar ways wasn't so bad after all.

Mail again and two regulars from Marion plus a package from Auntie.

Mail is essential but after reading it I always feel more lonesome than ever. The kids must be wonderful now—and Marion more lovely than ever.

Thursday, March 23, 1944

Still raining and very cold. Our stomach case is doing well so far. We have only the one so he's getting extra-special attention.

It seems this 10th Field outfit is deliberately making it unpleasant for us. Limiting our free time, unloading jobs on us that aren't ours, etc. We've had such good relations elsewhere I'm sure it isn't our fault.

Nothing doing on this front—still fighting bitterly at Cassino.

Saturday, March 25, 1944

More winter winds and cold. Our tents are about ready to take off in the breeze.

Very quiet—haven't had a patient in three days. From what the boys in the clearing station say there's nothing going on at the front and there's nothing in the wind right now.

Fighting is still grim at Cassino. We're getting the worst of that. We still have our backs to the wall at Anzio and on this front we haven't done a thing. The heavy air raids on Germany and the Russian advances are the only things from which you can gather hope right now.

Wednesday, March 29, 1944

Uneventful day—except the New Zealanders had to pull back from parts of Cassino (like we predicted)—otherwise no change in the war in Italy.

Fortunately the Russians are pressing hard. The guess here as of today is April 10th for the invasion, but I doubt it.

Heavy Jerry artillery barrage this afternoon but none came near us—just close enough to keep you concerned.

Sunday, April 2, 1944

Palm Sunday—but they use olive branches here in Italy. Beautiful day so we played two ball games this afternoon. No work for our shift.

Clyde Flood back at headquarters from Anzio and tells a pretty grim story of what goes on there. Five more of our group wounded when a bomb fell outside their tent. They're all dug in—even have the O.R.'s practically underground. As we played ball today we could look over on Jerry territory five miles away and see our own phosphorous shells break.

Monday, April 3, 1944

Broke our long string of workless days—got two cases in tonight and ours was really messed up. (Kidney, liver, small and large bowel.)

Colonel Forsee here this evening with the news that Sydoriak (here at 10th Field) is going home on rotation. Makes me sick to think that it will be months before my turn comes.

Got an oil burner tonight in place of our coal grate. Sounds peculiar—gas is rationed so closely in the States and we're burning it here in stoves. Costs $2.50 a gallon delivered to Italy. Stove costs 12.50 a day to run it. Rather expensive heat.

Tuesday, April 4, 1944

Had another case which kept us up half the night [case 54]. Work is still not heavy but it's increasing.

> Case 54. Diagnosis: Multiple shell fragment wounds—neck, left chest, left abdomen, both thighs, left knee. Abdominal wounds penetrating, perforating. Patient expired fourth post-operative day.

Wednesday, April 5, 1944

Had another real busy night—finished our last case at 11 this morning and I was just about finished.

This afternoon about 5 we had some Jerry shells landing awfully close. Came screaming in as if they were in the tent with you.

I'm dead tired tonight so I'm hoping we have a free night.

Thursday, April 6, 1944

Had a bad night as far as noise was concerned—Jerry shells started breaking near the bridge three or four miles away and they sounded as if they were in the tent with us.

Stars and Stripes show played over in the clearing station this afternoon.

Three regular letters from Marion today, all good ones—I'm really in love!

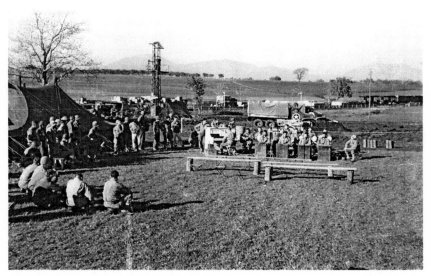

Stars and Stripes show at Carano.

Friday, April 7, 1944

Good Friday and we were more busy than ever. Had one fellow throw a massive hemorrhage from a neck wound—he died in two minutes. Kaplan had just started the anesthetic when the thing blew. Later found his carotid artery cut in half.

Understand Colonel Forsee finally went to Anzio. There's also some talk about replacing the teams up there—that means that we'll be certain to go up.

Saturday, April 8, 1944

Saw Bernadette of Lourdes this evening—very good. Case came in as it ended and we worked until 3 a.m. A fellow got slug in the rear that crossed his rectum into his belly.

Drove over in a truck to the 16th Evac and picked up Frank Hall's [Frank W. Hall, general surgeon][17] jeep. He's at headquarters and the jeep isn't on the books. Stopped in at the 11th Field and had supper. A platoon (Major Boylen's) is about to join the 85th Division Clearing Station on the coast road. Heard again that the 38th is replacing the 56th at the beachhead.

Sunday, April 9, 1944

Easter Sunday and it's been raining all day—but it doesn't make much difference. No place to go and no new clothes to wear. My man died this morning [case 54].

Didn't finish last night's case 'til 3:00 this morning and then was called again at 5:30 so I'm tired tonight. G. went into headquarters—colonel's back—says some of the boys up there are screaming for relief. I've got a feeling we're gonna make that beachhead yet.

No mail for me today—I feel lonely tonight—my second Easter away from home. Here's hoping I'm home next year.

Monday, April 10, 1944

Some changes are being made at Anzio—Swingle's team is leaving here tomorrow. Our turn will come soon—we can't help but get there soon. I guess it's only right that those fellows should be replaced. They've all been there since the beginning.

Work slowed up here today—had one case while we were on, which I did. Played a ball game this evening, which always helps me a great deal. The monotony of this place is killing.

Tuesday, April 11, 1944

No work today. 11th Field—Major Boylen's platoon—set up four miles away from us with the 85th Division Clearing Station. Frank Hall's team is there now and Taylor and Hunt to join them. They just came back from Anzio.

Heard an interesting story about the beachhead. As the 56th Evac was boarding L.S.T.s to leave the beach, Sally the German broadcaster was saying over her program that she hoped the 56th would get a good rest in Naples. And she welcomed the 38th Evac to the beachhead—all this they knew and right as it was happening.

Friday, April 21, 1944

Finally broke the mail silence yesterday and got a letter from Dad.

Enclosed a picture of Paulie and Joanie—I hardly knew them, they've grown so. (I'm sick of war!)

Had a case at 2 a.m.—first in quite awhile—mortar. Things very quiet here and Howard Snyder says they will be for a while. Side of the mountain ahead of us (10 miles?) was on fire tonight—phosphorous shells breaking. Flares were dropped over the river but heard no bombs.

Saturday, April 22, 1944

Anzio still calls—Ballantine got his orders and leaves tomorrow for the beachhead. We're due for a call someday soon. That load of first-class mail that came in yesterday supposedly was all a myth. I was certain I'd get mail today and didn't of course. Somehow these last few weeks I've been awfully low—here in Italy, at least, there's no sign of any headway being made. The beachhead has been open 90 days—all kinds of attempts at Cassino have failed. Now we're lining up for a try at this coastal area and I'm not so sure it won't fail—what I'd like to know is—when in the devil are they gonna open this second front?

Sunday, April 23, 1944

Ballantine and company left this afternoon for Anzio. No one here as yet to take his place—no business, however, so we really need no one. G. over at Major Boylen's this evening—he (Major B.) says we won't be going to Anzio—said he knew it to be a fact—so perhaps we're going to the 11th.

Monday, April 24, 1944

Moved across into the tent Ballantine left—it had floors. Got a case in at 4 p.m.—a badly "frapped" leg—really the worst soft-tissue wound I've seen [case 58]. Finished it at 9:30.

> Case 58. Operation started. Endotracheal ether. Large soft tissue wds. of thigh and leg widely debrided. Almost entire upper $1/3$ of femur shot away except the head and neck. Wd very extensive and penetrated to medial aspect of groin. Large comminuted comp fracture of knee. Condyles of femur almost destroyed. Large comp. com. fracture of tibia. S.V.G. dressings.

Planes over us in force tonight—Jerries attacking Naples. The ack-ack was pretty heavy. And to the front Jerry was throwing out artillery flares which lite the place up like high noon. Our guns were completely silent.

Wednesday, April 26, 1944

Had a good burn case come in this morning—80.9% of his body burned. Cook stove blew up. So far he's had 2,500 cc of plasma and it's still running [case 59]. Raining like hell all day—poured last night but we stayed dry. G. into Naples to the orange grove—he saw Sully and half the 2nd Aux there. News still very dull—from the quiet that prevails here I think the war has burned out. New moon is waxing—I'm hoping with all my might that something happens in the next two weeks.

Thursday, April 27, 1944

My burn case is much improved today—looks like he'll live.

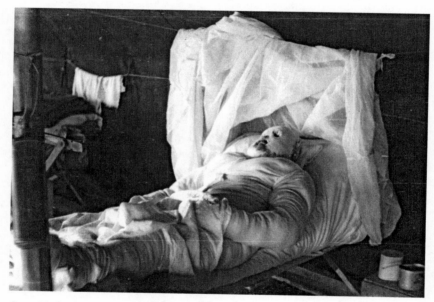

Case 59: burns over 80 percent of his body

No cases—everything as quiet as a church—nothing seems to happen—time just goes on—lots of time, and it's killing. These last few days have been the most difficult of any since I've been away from Marion. From Italy, at least, it looks like a long way from here 'til the end of the war—and it's very discouraging.

G. came in a little stewed last night—"blood rhubarb normal," he says.

Friday, April 28, 1944

The axe fell—we're Anzio bound. Colonel called—wanted to send us to 38th Evac but G. raised a stink so we'll probably go to 33rd Field. It's been a long time coming and now that it's definite I think I feel relieved.

Had a U.S.O. show here this afternoon—it's a mystery to me why they hauled them over here 'cause they were on the lousy side.

There's been a pretty heavy concentration of artillery fire tonight. Jerry kept flares over the bridge area for almost an hour and then kept throwing shells in.

Made the mail team today—first time in a long while.

Sunday, April 30, 1944

Another Sunday—that's the only sure way I know that time is passing. Had a flurry of cases in this evening—rifle grenade wounds. "Ted" [slang term for Germans, based on the Italian word for "German," *Tedesco*] put in a counterattack near Castleforte and took an O.P. [observation post] by surprise. Lots of artillery tonight. Leigh Haynes was up here this afternoon. He's been on the beachhead for a month—looks surprisingly good for what he went through. Beat a bomb to his foxhole by a split second.

Still no word about our Anzio trip.

Monday, May 1, 1944

Last night and early this morning turned out to be a busy period. Jerry put in more of an attack than we thought—he was stopped. At least he didn't get this far. Got a load of mail today—five regulars from Marion, so my day was a complete success.

Had sort of a dogfight—more of a chase—overhead today. A Spitfire chased a German observation plane around then out over the sea, shooting at him all the while—he missed.

Tuesday, May 2, 1944

Colonel Forsee here briefly this afternoon but didn't mention anything definite about Anzio. Said he'd need four teams. Told Major Plyler later that he was sorry but he'd have to take a few of the boys away from him here. We'll be included. He talked as if he expected things to happen real soon.

Wednesday, May 3, 1944

Rode down to the 36th General in Caserta today with our burn case—

T. [case 59]. Turned him over to Major Harvey Allen of the 12th General. He was favorably impressed with our treatment.

Everybody around here is sure something is going to happen Saturday or Sunday. Beautiful moonlight nights—good for love and war.

Thursday, May 4, 1944

Dance tonight at headquarters, particularly for the returning Anzio group. General Clark was invited but doubt if he'll appear.

No work at all—very little artillery but everything points to some action in a few days. We still haven't been told if we're gonna stay here or go to Anzio. The colonel works in mysterious ways.

(As each day passes by and adds to my foreign service, I spend more and more time thinking of home—Marion and the kids—it's been especially so today.)

3

Anzio and Rome

Friday, May 5, 1944

Got our call at 10:30 this morning. We're off to Anzio tomorrow—assigned to the 11th Evac. According to the boys who have returned from there, it's a pretty good deal.

I want to have this experience but as I desire it, it's only that I want it behind me. I would never ask for such a mission. So much can happen. But like everyone else I feel that it can't happen to me. It can't really because I have too much to live for.

Saturday, May 6, 1944

Gordon, Kaplan, and the enlisted men left today on an L.S.T. for the beachhead. No hospital ship sailed so I with my bevy of nurses will have to wait 'til tomorrow. Luther's team ordered back here today and they're going to the 11th Evac with us—also Lyman Brewer. We'll have a good bunch.

Sunday, May 7, 1944

Aboard U.S.S. *L.S.T. 76*

Mass and Communion this morning. All set to leave at 10:30 a.m. when orders for hospital ship again canceled. Finally sent off with Wolff's team at noon. Picked up Ken Lowry's [Kenneth F. Lowry, general surgeon] bunch at 52nd Station in Naples. As per usual, the 2nd Aux was bumming again—we loaded our equipment on partially loaded ammo trucks. Sailed from port above Naples at 4 p.m. and waited in center harbor 'til dark. Beautiful moon shining and we're sitting like ducks waiting to be shot. Capri just off to the left and Ischia ahead of us. Sailed away at about 9 p.m. Three L.S.T.s and a Liberty ship. Trog and Charlie spread their air mattress on the deck—I'll sleep between them. We're off to Anzio.

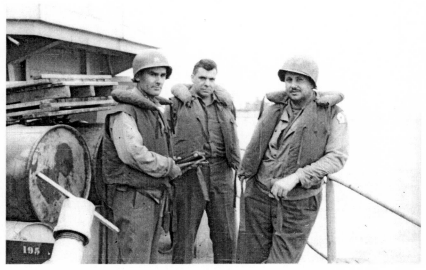

Charlie Westerfield, Luther Wolff, and Trogler Adkins aboard *LST 76*.

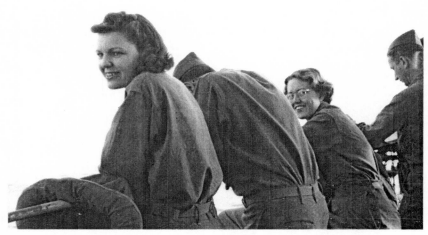

Nurses Lina Stratton and Frances Mosher aboard *LST 76*.

Monday, May 8, 1944

Anzio beachhead. Arrived in port at 10 a.m.—slow, rocky, uneventful trip. Few shells were falling in the water but were a safe distance from us. Anzio and Nettuno are nothing but a great series of shell holes—both towns have been demolished. Rode the loaded ammo truck out to the 11th Evac. All hospitals crowded into one area. Nice bunch of people here. We're living like moles but feel it safer. Would take a direct hit to get me. Saw the group at the 33rd Field and they are all down 10 feet. To see how all these hospitals are dug in is an amazing sight. How such a small area can hold so many people is a mystery to me.

(Paulie is six years old today—God bless and keep him.)

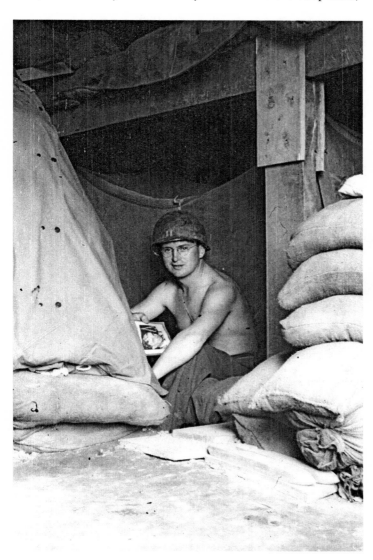

Kennedy in his "hoole" at Anzio.

Tuesday, May 9, 1944

Slept like a log last night even though the "Anzio Express" was riding the wind. That's a Jerry 210 that he rolls up at night—fires over our heads into Anzio and then retires. You hear the gun, then the whistle, followed by the boom. On call all day and on until 8 tomorrow. No work as yet. Just had an hour's air raid and it was a pip. I got caught on the way to the latrine but quickly retired to my tent. While the raid was on Jerry shelled. It's been over an hour but he's still shelling.[1] I'm gonna duck in bed and cover up my head—it's *no buono.*

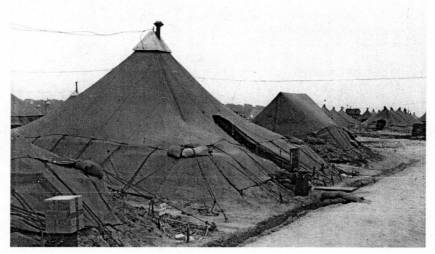

Kennedy's "flak shack," Eleventh Evacuation Hospital, Anzio

Wednesday, May 10, 1944

Still no work—Luther was on this 24 hours but had no cases either. There's no work of any sorts at any of the hospitals here. Had some ack-ack an hour ago and flak fell thru our tent. These flak shacks are handy things.

Thursday, May 11, 1944

Broke into the work column today. Had a belly case tonight [case 61]. We think we've got a pretty good arrangement here—we're gonna do nothing but the major stuff.

Case 61. Diagnosis: Penetrating wound right inguinal region (questionable peritoneal crossing). Fracture, compound, comminuted, right tibia and fibula, severe. Wound right ankle, lateral malleolus. Penetrating wound, medial surface left calf. Other superficial wounds.

Secret circular letter from General Alexander [Harold Rupert Leofric George Alexander, supreme Allied commander, Mediterranean] and General Clark read to all troops today saying in part that all was ready for a real push that with God's help would be successful.

Jerry threw in a pile of shells about 8 this evening and hit an ammo dump near Anzio. It's still burning fiercely. Now we're throwing out a real barrage—this may be the beginning.

Friday, May 12, 1944

The days are sunny and clear and fairly quiet, but when night comes all hell breaks loose. Last night I'd swear that each one of those shells was gonna land in the hole with me.

The attack on the main front started last night at 11 but nothing happened here. Supposedly they're going along all right down there. No work at all today. This sitting gets awfully tiresome and as always gives much too much time for thinking.

Saturday, May 13, 1944

It's 11:30 and I'm awfully sleepy but I don't think I can sleep through all this noise. A couple shells broke near us—sounded just as if they were under my bed. It's a very sickening noise—you hear the gun, then the whistle, and finally the burst.

On call but no work. They're still doing no fighting from this end. Not much news of what's going on down below. I'm sure they're having a tough time of it.

Sunday, May 14, 1944

I don't like to suggest at each entry that I'm fighting this war like an infantry soldier, but I promise you that our position here keeps you awfully uneasy. This morning about 5 a.m. "Ted" started throwing a few 170s in—about 30 rounds. They were only 100 yards away.

Took a tour of the beachhead today saw most everything but the front. Anzio and Nettuno were beautiful resort towns before the war but now they're both in ruins from shell fire. Got over to the 21st C.C.S. but missed Robby. Had tea there. Heard from Macfarlane of the 8th C.C.S. that the Americans are supposed to push out tonight.

Won $5 today from Wolff—I said the channel invasion wouldn't have taken place by 12 last night. Several sources quote tonight as the start of things from the beachhead. Supposedly things are going very well on main 5th Army front. Two air raids this evening—lots of ack-ack but no bombs. No work today.

The 2nd Aux group put a jackass in Swingle's tent—he's sort of a horse's ass and everybody thinks so.

Tuesday, May 16, 1944

Had another sleepless night—too much noise and too much stuff coming in—a brief air raid too. Such stuff isn't conducive to sound sleeping, at least not so far as I'm concerned.

Package from Marion with her picture and Ruthie's—both excellent and pleased me very much. Marion is really lovely.

Still making progress on main front. They're 2,000 yards across the Rapido—French doing well—now past Ausonia. No activity from the beachhead at all—everybody seems to expect it every day but nothing happens.

Wednesday, May 17, 1944

There's an air raid on now but it doesn't amount to much—however, I'm in my flak shack.

Still no work here. Heard today that it will be at least five more days before they push out from here.

Attended the first meeting of the Anzio Medical Society this evening at 33rd Field—Reeve Betts presiding.

News from main front seems to be good. South of the Liri River they have completely overrun the Gustav line and are approaching the Adolf Hitler line.

Thursday, May 18, 1944

Cassino was finally taken today. American units took Formia. The French got to Monticelli and the British took Cassino. The Adolf Hitler line is next. Still no activity on the beachhead.

Sunbath, exercises, and a shower—a big day. Mass over at the 94th Evac at 6:30 p.m. Stayed to a variety show there—very good.

Two letters from Marion today telling of Weiss's visit. I feel bad because he mentioned shells, etc.

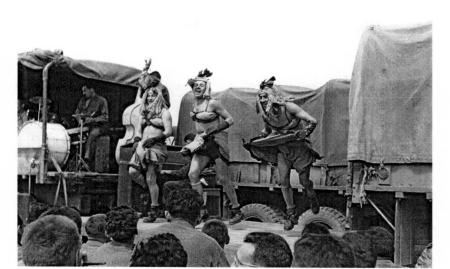

GI show: the "Andrews Sisters" at Ninety-Fourth Evac, Anzio

Friday, May 19, 1944

The beachhead remains comparatively quiet as far as work is concerned but actually there's lots of noise. The smoke screen blew away this afternoon and the Jerry-held mountains that rim us in were plainly visible. Makes you feel rather naked. Jerry is sort of looking down your throat.

Progress still continues and it looks like this may be the beginning of the end in Italy.

They opened a bar here tonight at the 11th Evac—rather nice but the drinks are terrible. Played ball this evening against the 3rd Medical Battalion.

Saturday, May 20, 1944

The news from the main front is all good. The Adolf Hitler line has been breached in several places. 5th Army only a few miles from Terracina—that's only 18 miles from us, so our day of liberation isn't far away. Heard tonight that the 16th Evac and 10th Field Hospital with nine of our teams are coming here. Talk now is that in 48 hours they're gonna push out of here. I'm sure they'll make it too. Luther's team had a case today but it wasn't much—our number still rests at one.

Sunday, May 21, 1944

Had quite a busy day—started operating at 9 this morning and didn't finish 'til 8 tonight. Had one die on us but he was awfully frapped up [case 63].

> Case 63. Diagnosis: SFW (shell fragment wounds) 1. Fracture, compound, comminuted right humerus into elbow joint. 2. Division brachial artery, right. 3. Multiple penetrating wounds, severe, buttocks, right; thigh, right; leg and foot, right; foot, left; thigh, left; entire lumbar region; chest, right. 4. Amputation, traumatic, 4th and 5th fingers, right hand, 2nd toe, left foot. 5. Shock, severe.

Had a beer ration here tonight in kegs and it was ice cold—tasted pretty good. Reminded me of the Nu Sig beer parties, but there was much less beer. Went over to 33rd Field after and had Yocky-Dockies. News pretty good today—Americans past Dondi—that's not far from us. Supposedly we're gonna lite out from here before the week's up. [Editor's note: the handwriting deteriorates as this entry progresses.]

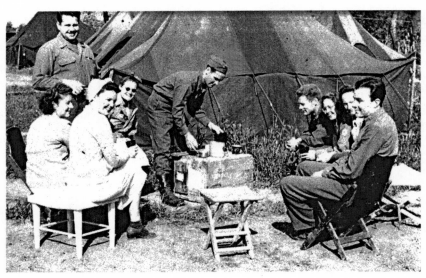

"Yocky-Docky" party

[Luther Wolff wrote,
    Yocky-Docky requires elucidation! One of the truly magnificent accomplishments of the medical department of the United States Army was the inclusion in the Table of Supplies of a five-

gallon drum of 95 percent ethyl alcohol, for sterilizing purposes.
. . . It became apparent at once that this fine, clean liquid had
great value, when properly diluted and flavored, in relieving ten-
sions and in making for splendid fellowship and conversation
in idle moments. . . . Various experiments were performed to
determine the best ingredients, but finally the following standard recipe became available because of its quickness and ease
of accomplishment. I do not know who coined the term "Yocky-
Docky," but it must have originated among the teams of the Second Auxiliary Surgical Group. . . . A standard prescription for
Yocky-Docky is as follows:

> Rx: 1 canteen, GI issue
> 1/3 canteen cup of 95 percent ethyl alcohol, GI issue
> 1/3 canteen cup of chlorinated water, GI issue
> 1 package of lemon powder, a constant ingredient of K
>   rations
> 2 lumps sugar, found in the K rations
> Sig: Misce

With the mixture properly prepared . . . the people assembled would sit in a circle and pass the cup in a clockwise direction. Refills were prepared by the host as needed. Sanitation was
quite well preserved by the alcohol.[2]]

Monday, May 22, 1944

Things are very quiet again today but supposedly tomorrow the attack
from the beachhead begins. Terracini was taken today so they have level
country to reach us up the Appian Way. There's a war going on right
now—you can actually see tracers firing from our own machine guns—
that's just a little too close. If all goes well this concentration camp should
be broken up very soon and soon we shall see Rome. But then where to?

Tuesday, May 23, 1944

This morning at dawn the beachhead forces struck. Took Cisterna by
noon and cut Highway 7. Casualties are heavy, however. We've had over
200 surgical admissions. We did only seven cases all day but they were
all field hospital cases. It's 12 midnight and we go to bed 'til 7 a.m. The
artillery barrage wasn't awfully heavy this morning but there was lots of
air activity. Jerry didn't stop the Anzio Express, however—he laid them
in awfully close tonight.

Six 2nd Aux teams came up today. 16th Evac and 10th Field coming tomorrow.

(Got a cute picture of Ruthie—she's a dream.)

Wednesday, May 24, 1944

It's 7 p.m. and we're going to bed until 1 a.m. Worked from 7 this morning. We still have 170 cases waiting operation and a large number of the minor wounded have been evacuated to Naples. The casualties are heavy and every hospital on the beachhead is full. It's hard to get any news of how things are going—all right, we guess and hope. Jerry has been frapping them frequently—last night I just hung onto the bed and prayed. I hope that this attempt liberates the beachhead. Box from Marion today—good snacks.

Thursday, May 25, 1944

9 p.m. and I'm heading for bed. Started this morning at 1 a.m. and have worked continuously until now—did five bellies, among other things. Last one died suddenly on the table.

5th Army main forces and the beachhead forces met today. Progress seems to be good (but the Anzio Express still rides). At the passing of the first shell I wake up with a start and hear every one after that. I'm awfully tired tonight—so tired I'll have a hard time sleeping—my feet hurt.

Friday, May 26, 1944

It's 10 p.m. and I'm just getting in bed. We go back on at 1:30 a.m. so I've little time to sleep. Had most of the work cleaned up but it started coming in again this evening. Situation is good. Route 7 is open to Naples. Major Plyler (10th Field) here this evening—he drove up today. Troops are 20 miles from Rome and at the rate they're going they'll be there in a week. 33rd Field is moving out tomorrow and I sorta wish we were with them. I like to keep moving. Nice letters from Marion—more pictures—she's a darling and oh, how I'd like to see her.

Saturday, May 27, 1944

Went to work this morning at 1 a.m. and we've been going all day—it's now five of 11 and we're going to bed. Had a lot of excellent cases and did OK by them. Colonel Wilson and Colonel Taber have been very generous in their praise of our team. We have worked long hours and have done a lot. Colonel Taber told us tonight that he told General Martin what a wonderful job we've done.

Had a real air raid here last night at 12:00—they really rocked us. Casualties have dropped off and the progress is now excellent. We'll be in Rome soon, I'll bet.

Sunday, May 28, 1944

On at 7 a.m. Had a good sleep except for a couple hours. There was a real air raid and things were so noisy you couldn't hear yourself think. Did four good belly cases—all were frapped up. Our other cases are doing very nicely, with few exceptions. We're getting a lot of good cases but I'm getting more tired all the time—my feet hurt and my eyes are half closed—and the cases still come rolling in. Got several Jerries—both nice fellows and very appreciative. Teams at other hospitals here not doing half as much. Had one case today that was wounded four miles from Rome.

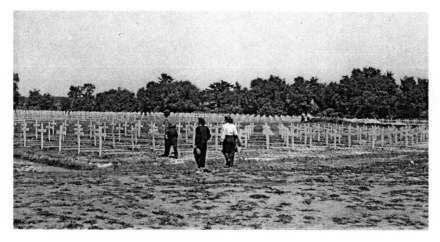

American cemetery at Anzio.

Monday, May 29, 1944

Still working, though the pressure seems to be letting up. Had more good abdominal and chest cases today. We've done 22 bellies in five days—real labor. Platoon of 10th Field went out today to replace the 33rd Field. VI Corps reorganizing for something but nobody seems to know what for.

Colonel Forsee here this evening. Told us rotation was off but that furloughs of a month would start soon—then return overseas. Progress has been slowed a little—can't seem to find out definitely where the line is. Everybody is "Rome hungry."

Tuesday, May 30, 1944

Got in bed today after noon meal—just going back to work now at 11:30 p.m.—I didn't sleep worth a damn—can't in the daytime. I'll be an old man if this thing keeps up much longer. And according to all rumors they're getting ready to start another push very soon for Rome. Right now I need a rest and not more work. There are all sorts of speculations as to what will happen to the 2nd Aux when Rome falls—southern France, England, Yugoslavia, and India have all been mentioned—my guess is England.

Wednesday, May 31, 1944

We've changed hours again—for the tenth time—8 p.m. to 8 a.m. now. Finished up at 3:00 this afternoon and we're going back at it now—it's 8 p.m. I don't think the Russian salt mines were ever any worse than this. There's another push on and we're getting another load—200 cases behind now. There are four field hospital platoons out now—two of the 33rd and two of the 10th, so we'll be cut down on the major cases.

Thursday, June 1, 1944

Progress has been quite good but the casualties have been high. We're not seeing the worst cases now 'cause the field hospitals have jumped ahead. Expect we'll be going to one of them soon. Doing simple debridements here these past couple days and they are monotonous and boring.

Friday, June 2, 1944

Had a fairly good sleep but it's never as restful as what you get at night. We'll be off this night tour in another week. At the rate things are moving now I think they'll be in Rome in a week. They're at the Alban hills and at some points nothing stands between them and Rome—except a few Jerries.

  Not much work tonight—mostly minor stuff. Another field hospital platoon went out this evening. Hope we get assigned soon. Had a few snaps of Ruthie today—she's a wonderful baby.

Saturday, June 3, 1944

The shock ward was empty for the first time this morning—seems queer not being loaded with casualties. Luther had word this morning that his team was gonna leave to join the 11th F.H. without us—but tonight at 7:30 we got orders to leave too. Packed in half an hour, said our good-byes, and set out for a place near Cori. Staying here tonight with the 95th Evac. Harry Borsuk here—platoon leader—hospital to be beyond Valmontone about 15 miles from Rome on Highway 6. Came through Cisterna—worst destruction I've seen yet. There's nothing standing. We're back in a field hospital and on our way to Rome. I'm happier when we're moving—moving toward home!

Sunday, June 4, 1944

Up at 6:30 (good night's rest)—had pancakes, then set out in a weapons carrier for our new site. The number of wrecked Jerry vehicles, guns, etc. is a mute tribute to the work of our aircraft. The roads were just covered with wrecks—large tanks with 88s pointing dumbly into the ground—a few 170s (Anzio Express) that looked awfully powerful but now appeared to be dead. Valmontone, Cori, and Labico are all shot up and have nothing left.

Dead horses stinking—even the smell of rotting human flesh filtering through occasionally. We're set up near Palestrina on Highway 6 with the 3rd Division Clearing Station. Work is pouring in already—rearguard action, the boys say. "Jerry is on the run" and some of our troops are on the outskirts of *Rome.*

Monday, June 5, 1944

Business it seems to follow us wherever we go. Cases galore—more than we could handle. We're the most forward field hospital now. Brought in three new teams to help out and they were very welcome. Brinker, Lowry, and Cantlon [Edwin L. Cantlon, general surgeon]. Rome is in our hands—was yesterday—and the troops are beyond. Evidently Jerry intends to keep running for a while. Tanks have been going by here all day in one steady stream—last night they rumbled by in countless numbers. I'm sure somebody is gonna be impressed by them very soon. The war is moving fast—good—I want it that way—I want to get home.

Tuesday, June 6, 1944

Rome

Up early, got our work done (off call for once), and a group of us headed for Rome. I was anxious. The mark of the war looks fresh upon the country that leads to Rome—burned-out tanks, guns, etc. Dead horses—and people streaming back to their homes.

Rome seems to be a beautiful city. Little destruction, nice-looking

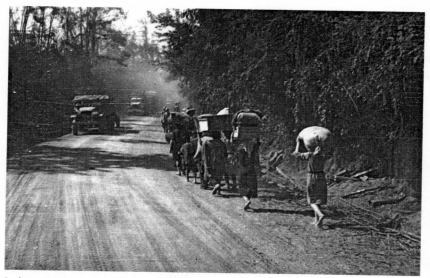

Italian civilians returning to their homes after the fall of Rome.

people—much cleaner than the more southern Italians—more like a city in the States. Saw St. Peter's and knelt by the Tomb of St. Peter.

It's a magnificent church, strong and tall, and it suggests Catholicism—enduring. Crossed the Tiber, saw the Coliseum and Roman Forum. This was the Rome we were waiting for.

(Incidentally, the second front opened today, but we saw Rome.)

[The "incidental" second front was nothing less than Operation Overlord, the cross-channel invasion of France at Normandy, involving almost sixty-five hundred naval craft and five Allied divisions. Eventually, more than one hundred divisions were to pass through Normandy on their way to the very heart of Germany and to the ultimate destruction of the Third Reich.]

Wednesday, June 7, 1944

Worked from 1 a.m. to 6, then to bed for an hour. Little work coming in—the 94th Evac and 10th Field open ahead of us. Went into Rome again at 1:00 and did some shopping. Prices haven't started to hit the sky as yet but they will shortly. Already the people seem to have accepted the troops—not so much cheering, etc., but Rome is alive with eager soldiers. A couple truckloads of prisoners drove past us in town—they got a poor reception from the people. Got some pictures of them.

Thursday, June 8, 1944

Did very little of anything and enjoyed it—after working so hard, having nothing to do is a pleasure for a while. Got the car from the C.O. and went in search of our laundry this morning—got over to Palestrina. It's just another frapped-up town. Built a shower this afternoon and then had a good bath—very good shower it is.

The three teams that joined us here were moved on today to a platoon of the 10th Field Hospital going above Rome—Civitavecchia, a port 40 miles above Rome fell today. We're really moving fast. Rumor today says II Corps is pulling out to train for amphibious landing!!

Friday, June 9, 1944

Went into Rome early this morning and spent the whole day—looking. Searched some stores for some Chanel no. 5 but didn't see any. Saw the Pantheon, built in 127 B.C. Had dinner at the Excelsior Hotel—a very beautiful place—to be an officers' rest camp. The hotels are on a hill in a very pretty part of town. Got a ride out to the Catacombs on Appia Antica. Saw thru a part of them and was impressed with my own insignificant part in time.

Climbed all around the Coliseum taking pictures. Then to the Roman Forum and Senate and then back home—tired out.

Saturday, June 10, 1944

A beautiful lazy day in the sun. Had nothing to do but loaf. Developed some of the pictures I've taken and they turned out all right. This loafing feels pretty good for a change. The 2nd Aux is moving in behind the Vatican. Rumor is quite prevalent that the American troops are pulling out of Italy; getting ready for another amphibious operation—southern France.

Tuesday, June 13, 1944

Evacuated all patients this morning to the 38th Evac in Rome. Colonel here this afternoon from 5th Army headquarters at Anzio. We're to move with this platoon of the 11th Field tomorrow above Rome—how far is a question. It seems the line is moving so fast that field hospitals, let alone evacs, can't keep up. We're supposed to move out of here at 2:30 a.m.—they've routed us around about so we're just gonna lose the convoy and go into our headquarters for breakfast.

There's been a change in the platoon since Major Boylen left—it's not too good now.

Wednesday, June 14, 1944

Up at 2:30 a.m. to move with 11th Field (unnecessary). We left the convoy, much to Borsuk's disgust, and went to our headquarters in Rome. They're well set up behind the Vatican in very pretty park. Would like to have stayed there for a while. Drove north over Route 1—coast road—thru Civitavecchia, Tarquinia, Montalto, to Orbetello. We're with the 2nd Platoon of the 33rd Field for a while. We are again abreast of the artillery, such as it is. Much of the country between here and Rome shows little evidence of war—except for bombed-out bridges, etc. Civitavecchia is being used as a port already and the harbor was filled with shipping. The Anzio Express was there. Stepped in and did two cases before 12 midnight. One division in the line—the 36th.

Thursday, June 15, 1944

A big gun just off to our left kept booming away all night—but today the war has gone on and left us. The casualties stopped as suddenly, so we were free all day. Drove out to the island—Argentano and to the port at its northern end—San Stefano. The Germans left five days ago and destroyed everything else that American bombs hadn't ruined. The town and road to it were shambles. Some fishermen rowed us across the bay— took a picture of one fellow who helped six American flyers escape to Sardinia—he rowed them across in a small boat.

Saw a truck on the way back that five minutes before ran thru a minefield—hit five mines. Three men in truck killed!

Saturday, June 17, 1944

Moving day again—Wolff, Jarvis, and our team moved 18 miles up the road (five miles south of Grosetto) to join the 2nd Platoon of the 11th Field (Joe Barnard). We're back alongside the guns and they're banging away right now.

Casualties, however, are light. Rained on the way up here and we got slightly soaked.

Got some mail before we left the 33rd Field and I made a good haul—pictures et al.—but boy, it makes me lonely.

Sunday, June 18, 1944

Had a case first thing this morning—fellow was mortally wounded, I'm afraid [case 131].

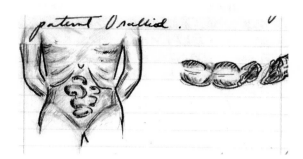

Case 131

Case 131. C. F. M. Pvt. 6956469 Age 22 B'try B. 916 F.A. Bn.
Injured 0545 hrs. 18 June 44 Shell fragment.
Injured near Groseto, Italy. He was picked up in a jeep given
a half (½) gr. of morphine and was brought to Field Hosp
directly.
11th Field Hosp. 0715 hrs.
gen'l condition poor. B.P. 150/68 P 70 perspiring freely. four
feet of small bowel had eviscerated thru wound.
Pre op Rx. 0715 1 unit plasma. 0730 hrs. 2nd unit of plasma
B.P. 120/70 P 72 0745 hrs. B.P. 120/70 P 76 Atropine SO4
gr 1/75

Operation: Endotracheal ether & O2 500 cc blood started.
Left rectus incision made to include wd. of entrance. Small bowel
previously cleansed with saline. Jejunum had been transected in
several places one 4" from ligament of Treitz. Small bowel resection done—end to end anastomoses. Left half of transverse colon
and proximal portion of descending colon badly torn. Interven-
ing small portion of splenic flexure removed. and free ends of
colon brought as a double barrel colostomy thru left stab wd. F.B.
had penetrated retroperitoneally transecting the kidney. Kidney
removed transperitoneally. Two penrose cigarette drains led thru
flank stab wound to kidney bed. There was a considerable amount
of corn and powdered eggs free in the peritoneal cavity. Feces also
free in peritoneal cavity. Abdomen closed in layers. T.&T. retention sutures. 10 gms. sulfanilamide into peritoneal cavity. 5 gms.
sulf. into kidney bed. 2000 cc blood during operation. Two veins
employed. Operation ended. B.P. 80/40. During operation B.P.
had fallen to 0 and pulse was nil but patient rallied.

(That was the Britishers' famous saying at 8th C.C.S.—their patients all get well unless they're mortally wounded.) Rained like hell last night— thundered and lots of lightning and much artillery. Can see the guns from here. They're fighting five miles beyond Grosetto. 8th Evac moved in next door, so our work won't be too heavy. Headquarters of 11th Field also moved up. No room ahead for a field hospital as yet.

Meant to note that from our position here we can see the island of Elba where Napoleon spent 10 months.

Monday, June 19, 1944

A lazy day—didn't get a case. (Actually don't care if we never did another.) Drove up the road to the gun emplacements—155s—our Long Toms. They were getting ready to fire a mission—last night they fired continuously. Had word the Jerries were getting ready to pull out so they were getting set to blast them. Miss Price (2nd Aux chief nurse) and Ben Schneiderman were here this evening. Said F.D.R. was supposed to be in Rome—Grand Hotel. Also German envoys were supposed to be in the Vatican. Rumors like these get your hopes high but nothing ever happens.

Tuesday, June 20, 1944

There's always something coming along to make life uncomfortable. Brott [Clarence R. Brott, assistant general surgeon][3] drove back to the 94th today and brought back the rumor that the colonel was out look- ing for volunteers. Sure enough, he drove in here this evening and hinted around that something was coming up. Said he wanted us to sleep on it— he'd see us in the morning. Well, we won't volunteer but I'm sure we're slated to go wherever it is.

Wednesday, June 21, 1944

Colonel Forsee in his very indirect way warned us about a new webfoot operation that's coming up soon. We're on his list to go. Iovine [Vincent M. Iovine, general surgeon] and Wolff set too. Southern France or Yugo- slavia is the destination. Now more stew for a while. Drove up to Gro- setto and looked around. Pretty church there—these people, it seems, put everything they have into the building of beautiful churches. The farm- ing country between there and the sea is really beautiful. We went from farmhouse to farmhouse buying eggs. Got three dozen at 5¢ apiece. They haven't learned as yet what eggs are selling for. The roads leading down to the sea had all been heavily mined. Engineers were digging them up yesterday.

Saturday, June 24, 1944

It's pitch black and the guns are shaking the ground once again. We moved some 30 miles and are back with the war again—near Follonica. This time it seems we moved just a little too close. On the way here we passed battalion aid stations, mortar patrols on the march—had to ford a couple streams across which the engineers hadn't had time to fix bridges. It's funny to see the infantry soldiers react to seeing nurses this far forward—one of them just stood with his hands on his hips and said, "I'll be damned."

Got mail this morning—lots from Marion.

I meant to note that we moved the army way. Got orders at 6:00 this evening.

Sunday, June 25, 1944

Had a noisy night but no work came in. They made their attack at 12:00 but Jerry wasn't there to greet them. Drove into Follonica this afternoon. According to B.B.C. this morning it's still in German hands. Streets and beaches here were heavily mined—watched engineers digging them up. Some of the fields outside still had signs in German marking the mined areas. They pulled out very quickly around here. Got seven cases in this evening and we did three of them. Two of those cases were bilateral amputations. One kid was 19 years old.

Very quiet here—once more the war has moved off and left us.

Monday, June 26, 1944

2nd Platoon has jumped us again so our work is finished, I guess. The 111th Clearing is closing as the 36th is pulling out of the line. They're going to Salerno for amphibious training. I talked with a litter bearer over there tonight who was captured at Velletri and then escaped 10 days later at Originale, 30 miles north of Rome. He told me some interesting stories—poor food, hardly any at all. Germans using horses to draw some of their artillery, shortage of gas, etc. He and his friend hid in a cave—hid in cellars of Eyeties and finally got away.

Did no work at all today and probably will do no more here.

Tuesday, June 27, 1944

Another platoon going out tomorrow so we'll be moving again. We're having very short stays: doing a minimum amount of work, seeing a maximum of country.

Cherbourg fell today. That means they've got a large port in France now, which will facilitate things very much.

Sullivan came in today—he had just been out looking for a site for headquarters. They're moving up from Rome. Most important—he brought a load of mail and I got eight letters from Marion—(a good day). I've known Marion a long time now, but I'm just as much in love with her as ever. I still get a thrill when I think of her.

Wednesday, June 28, 1944

Got orders to move up (G.S. [General Surgery] 15 and 6) to a clearing station (54th Medical Battalion) supporting the 1st Armored Division and a combat team of the 91st Division. Drove thru Massa Marittima to just beyond Prata below Gabellino crossroads. It was an advance of 21 miles over pretty rugged mountainous country. Never saw so many dead horses along the road. Lots of Jerry equipment too—they ran thru here only two days ago. We didn't see a sign of Yanks for miles, and a couple times shells hit fairly close (we were going parallel to the front). It's just a little uneasy at such times. We set up in a field right in the middle of a battery of 155s—fortunately they were about to pull out.

This medical outfit isn't equipped to do surgery but we're supposed to do it.

Thursday, June 29, 1944

Business not very rushing even though we did make a good hop. The front has moved again, and according to one ambulance driver we're 50 miles behind again. The 33rd Field Hospital Unit II moved in this afternoon so we'll operate with them.

Country hereabouts is absolutely beautiful—and very hot too. I walked up the road away to the 1st Armored C.P. [Command Post]— never saw so much activity. I wonder if they all knew what they were doing. I am constantly amazed at the amount of equipment we have there—you just can't imagine it could ever be possible.

Friday, June 30, 1944

Got word this morning that we move again tomorrow. After this I don't think it will even be worthwhile to take my hat off. Worked practically all day. Did one case at the 54th Medical Battalion last night—like working on the kitchen table, but not too bad.

According to the word we've had, the Jerries are going back so fast now they're being caught in their own minefields—*Achtung Minen!* signs all over the place.

Saturday, July 1, 1944

Tore down right after breakfast and set out for our new area. Went about 20 miles to a point near Montingegnoli—about five miles short of area, an M.P. stopped us and told us we were in artillery range—and as it turned out he was quite right. The 155s are now behind us. We're set up in a grove along a cool stream—very nice. The roads are dusty and yesterday it was hot so first thing we did was to take a dip, and what a delight it was.

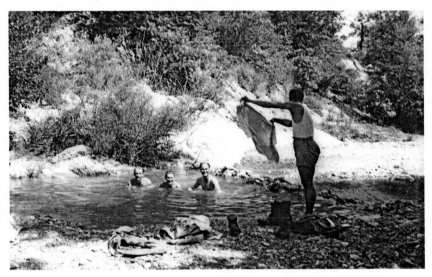

Second Aux officers taking a dip in the brook at the camp near Montingegnoli.

An hour after we were set up, the division surgeon came by and said we wouldn't open—we were gonna move again. Came back in another hour to say we'd work here. Had one real case tonight. It's 60 miles from here to an evac—this fellow would have died if he had to make that trip [case 136].

Case 136. Diagnosis: Fracture, skull, basal, severe 2) Rupture traumatic, bladder, extra peritoneal, severe. 3) F.C.C. sacro-iliac, rt., severe 4) Rupture, traumatic, cecum 5) Fracture dislocation, severe, left ankle. 6) Wds, multiple, leg, tr. pen severe, all incurred when vehicle hit land mine at 0230 hrs. 30 June 44 near Monte Castella, Italy.

Post-op: Returned to ward in fair condition.

Sunday, July 2, 1944

Did one case during the night—only had two teams here until this afternoon when Ballantine arrived so it keeps you busy—and fresh out of sleep. We are experiencing now the worst food that we've met so far, and probably this is the worst hospital we've been with. Colonel Bennett—C.O. (Someday I hope to be able to tell him.) Somebody mentioned to him that the food was pretty poor and he jumped down their throat, saying nobody could criticize his hospital.

(Few shells landed over the hill from us this morning—too close.)

Monday, July 3, 1944

Up at 2:30 a.m. to do a case—got back in bed at 5 a.m. so tonight I'm tired—didn't sleep all day. There seems to be a bottleneck about 15 miles up the road that they're having a time clearing. The tanks just go sailing up the road until suddenly the lead tank is blown off the road by a concealed 88. An Arm'd [armored division] chaplain here yesterday said they've had fairly heavy tank casualties, but casualties in men haven't been heavy here. Siena fell to the French today. They had no opposition there.

No word of moving yet. Our next area is still under mortar fire.

Tuesday, July 4, 1944

Just the ordinary amount of artillery even though it was the 4th. But there were other kinds of fireworks and with a bark that has at least some bite. Michaels here from headquarters recalling teams for the coming webfoot operation. We are on it and on the first group. G.S. 15 [Luther Wolff's team] not recalled. I hope I can write the finish as I do the beginning. Hospital moving out tomorrow. Sienna and beyond in our hands. They say they expect Florence tomorrow or soon, but there's still a pocket to our left by six miles that's holding out.

Few of the nurses on a tour of the country yesterday got some meat—steaks—so last evening we had a charcoal fire all set to grill the meat. It turned out to be horsemeat—terrible.

Wednesday, July 5, 1944

Up for an early breakfast—hospital moving about 14 miles up the road while we waited for trucks from headquarters. Finally got off to headquarters by 2 a.m. and arrived here at 6, just in time for a turkey dinner, which was excellent. Headquarters set up five miles north of Follonica. Very nice area. Officers' Club with iced drinks and all.

Many teams here getting ready for the invasion—some indefinite but we've already been told we're going. Southern France is everybody's guess. 22 teams going so it must be a big operation. Now I've got this to sweat out until I'm safe in whatever country we're headed toward.

Thursday, July 6, 1944

Headquarters is close to being a rest camp and I must say is enjoyable (quite an admission to make about 2nd Aux headquarters). They opened a beach a couple miles from here and I spent all afternoon there—very nice. Elba seems to be only a mile or so away (actually it's seven miles). Few more teams back today—evidently this is gonna be a big affair.

Movie here this evening, which was excellent—first one I've seen in days.

Friday, July 7, 1944

Left headquarters at 9:30 a.m. on the spur of the moment for Rome. Tony Emmi in to buy liquor and Jim Mason going to the 6th General. Arrived in Rome at 3 p.m. and found a room with an Italian family at Via Muzio Clementi and Via Pietro Corsa. Tony immediately took off and I was left to Rome (about). Walked my feet off, too, just looking. Had ice cream at the Red Cross, then ate dinner at Broadway Bill's, and later (8:30) ate again with my Italian friends. They had a surprisingly good meal. Steak and potatoes and a fresh green salad. They seemed quite amused at me and through one of them that could talk English they asked me a thousand questions.

Saturday, July 8, 1944

Up at 8:30. Breakfast consisted of one roll and a cup of awful coffee (chicory). Walked over to St. Peter's and hired a guide all by my lonesome. Spent a couple hours just looking and listening. Went over to the Vatican entrance then and waited for an hour before the Swiss Guards let us in. They are big, nice-looking fellows dressed in royal-blue hose pants and shirt to match—a black tam and black shoes. I climbed a thousand steps to get to the room where the audience was to be held. Large room highly decorated but in good taste. Had a good seat only 10 or 15 feet from the pope's throne. Pope was carried in on a chair—dressed in white robe with white skullcap. He is certainly a gracious person and made a profound impression on all. He spoke briefly in English and then in French, saying that all true hope and peace comes in living close to God. Afterward he stepped down from his throne and talked with some officers, asking them where they were from—what army they were in, etc. I edged my way in and held his hand and knelt and kissed his ring. I was thrilled and can't really say what I felt. He said that thru each of us he sent his blessing back to our loved ones overseas.

Sunday, July 9, 1944

This was an extra day in Rome. We planned on leaving this morning but the enlisted man who came with us didn't return from visiting his grandparents (he had never seen them). Went to Mass this morning in a little church just around the corner. You get a peculiar feeling attending Mass in an Italian church—you can't help but get the idea that no one there knows just what is going on—people coming and going—some sitting; some standing—only a few kneeling. Walked up to the Red Cross for a cup of coffee and wrote some letters and then went on to Broadway Bill's (G.I. joint) for dinner. Walked about some more and then back for a good supper with my Italian friends. We sat and thru one we all talked until bedtime.

Monday, July 10, 1944

Up early and finally got away from Rome at 9 a.m. Had the back of the weapons carrier full of glasses, chairs, tables, and cognac so that we jingled with every bounce. Back here at 3 p.m. Had three packages waiting for me and one of them had two cans of beer in it—very good. No new rumors on our moving, but the story is we're going by boat to Naples from Piombino. (Much better than by truck.)

4

Operation Dragoon and the Pursuit up the Valley of the Rhone

Tuesday, July 11, 1944

Mail would be scarce at a time like this! There are probably a thousand things I should say—should write—but better to be an optimist, I believe. (I'm sure everything will come out all right.) Repacked my stuff for the tenth time today, trying to fit too much into too little space. Rolled all my bulk film and fixed it in a waterproof package just in case we get dunked. Seems somebody in the outfit talked too much about this procedure to someone in an official capacity, so this evening we were all firmly warned about keeping our mouths shut.

Thursday, July 13, 1944

Tore down everything this morning got all packed and as per usual we hurried to wait. Went by truck to Piombino and there boarded the filthiest Liberty ship in circulation: the *William B. Floyd*. Still unloading rations so we won't sail until tomorrow morning at 6:30. Few of the majors have rooms but the majority of us are down in one hatch sleeping on Bradford frames and hot as hell. We're going to Naples supposedly to stage a while but oh, how I wish this boat were sailing for home.

Friday, July 14, 1944

Sailed from Piombino this morning at 6:30—with two other Liberty ships and a little protection. Beautiful day, water smooth and real blue—very pleasant. (What a wonderful time Marion and I could have on a nice boat here.) Passed Monte Cristo Island at noon. There are some 700 on board and this tub is supposed to carry 45 passengers so we're really crowded. Soldiers and officers too are stretched out all over the place, in the lifeboats, on the hatches, and all over. Food isn't too bad but we have to eat in five shifts and it takes a little while.

129

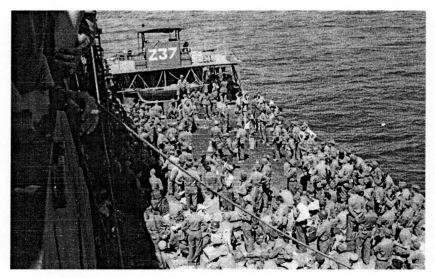

Aboard the *William B. Floyd*

Saturday, July 15, 1944

Pulled into Civitavecchia this afternoon and we're staying here all night to join a convoy for Naples tomorrow. Been thru this town twice previously on land and it's all knocked to hell—it was the port of Rome once but now is a port of war, but soon the war will leave it—to a new birth.

Sunday, July 16, 1944

Pulled out of C last night and arrived in the harbor of Naples at 12 noon and there we've sat ever since. This place is loaded with freighters and few personnel vessels. One freighter has a locomotive on its deck. Everybody is getting very restless—seems like we've been on here an age. The ship is filthier than ever and the plumbing is beginning to go. Tonight high up in the pile of life rafts we had a Yocky-Docky party 'til we ran out of things. Lot of drinking going on in "Berget's Din" [Berget H. Blocksom Jr., general surgeon]—a madhouse. This place I'm sleeping in is a real den.

Monday, July 17, 1944

Last night was the worst yet. I haven't had any real sleep in days. 200 of us are crowded down in hatch 3—a poker game goes 'til all hours in one corner. They play poker at the foot of my bed 'til dawn—a pair of nines

was the last hand early this morning. Then at 3 a.m. we had an air raid—
what excitement.

There's a hatch open right above us and in the shooting and noise
a soldier on deck fell thru the hatch, hit me in the head in passing, then
landed on my glasses and broke them. Finally got off the boat at 3 p.m.
Our trucks met us and we drove right out to Sparanise. We're going with
the 11th Field and we're with our favorite division. (Father's Day card
waiting here for me—I'm more lonesome than ever.)

Tuesday, July 18, 1944

Had a good night's rest. Breakfast with Plyler over at the 10th Field, then
into Naples. Put an order in for my glasses, then had dinner at the 45th
General.

Naples is a million miles from the war, as far as I could see. Suntans
all over the place, summer blouses, etc. I guess base sections are necessary, but they're certainly unpopular.

Wednesday, July 19, 1944

Spent most of the morning moving across the road to the 11th Field Hospital area. Getting rather expert at this tent-pitching business. A gang of
us took a truck and drove up to Cassino, or rather what was Cassino.
Nothing more than a disorganized rock pile. I have never seen such complete destruction. After being so close to it for so long it was interesting
to finally see it. It's easy now to understand how the Jerries were able to
hold out for so long.

Thursday, July 20, 1944

Into Naples again first thing. Took my radio to try and have it fixed—on
the blink again—but had no success. Got my glasses and then had lunch
at the 21st General. Had a bacon, lettuce, and tomato sandwich with
a chocolate malted milk. Went back downtown and had two ice-cold
Cokes at the P.X. Went up to the Allied Officers' Club then and had dinner—it's in the old Orange Club high up on a hill overlooking the Bay of
Napoli—very nice terraces, etc.—a beautiful place. Home by 10 and to
bed. No news on coming event.

Friday, July 21, 1944

Started again to get my radio fixed but only got word of where the unit
is—instead I visited Russell in Caserta at the 8th General Dispensary.
It's bad for me to go back and see such places—see how they're living

and eating; not knowing a thing about what war feels like and tastes like. Majors—colonels—generals all dressed up with their pants pressed. There's so damn much injustice that it's sickening—there's no war for them—.

Nothing new on our purpose.

B.B.C. news of unrest in German Army and attempt on Hitler's life is all good news.

[On July 20, Colonel Claus von Stauffenberg, a highly decorated veteran who had been severely wounded in action in Tunisia, succeeded in detonating a bomb in the conference room of Hitler's retreat at Rastenburg in eastern Prussia. Although the bomb killed or mutilated a number of Hitler's staff, Hitler himself emerged with only minor injuries. The assassination of Hitler was supposed to set in motion a conspiracy to seize control of the government and the army and depose the Nazi regime. The conspirators had vaguely formed and changing concepts of then seeking some kind of peace agreement with the western Allies.

Intensely patriotic, Stauffenberg had become convinced that Hitler was leading Germany to ruin—as indeed he was—and that he had to be stopped. To this end he joined a number of army officers, apparently including Rommel, in an attempt to overthrow the regime. The plot was probably doomed to failure from the start. On the day, the need for precise timing, decisive action, and the manipulation of many ponderous moving parts collided with human frailty, as some of the plotters carefully and continually tested the winds rather than fulfilling their assignments as planned. Perhaps most damaging, the indispensable, decisive, and fully committed Stauffenberg spent the crucial early hours of the implementation of the insurrection isolated and out of touch during his long, slow flight back from Rastenburg to Berlin, only to discover upon arrival that virtually nothing had been accomplished. On top of this, with the news that Hitler had survived (widely disseminated because the rebels inexplicably failed to silence the national radio network), the insurrection crumbled. Stauffenberg and three of his fellow conspirators were shot that very evening, spared the gruesome and barbaric treatment later visited by Hitler upon others who were implicated in the plot. As he stood before the firing squad, Stauffenberg cried out his last words: "Long live our sacred Germany."[1]

As for Hitler, he viewed his miraculous escape from all but the most trivial of injuries and the failure of the plot as proof of the righteousness of his cause: "I regard this as a confirmation of the task imposed upon me by Providence."[2]]

Sunday, July 23, 1944

Ruthie is a year old today and still I haven't seen her. I feel certain that the time isn't too far away when I'll be home and with all my family again—I can't help feeling that song—"You'll Be So Nice to Come Home To"—was written for me.

> Dearest Ruthie,
>
> It hardly seems possible that my little girl is already a year old. It seems in many ways a very short time since I read in the *Stars and Stripes* while I was in Sousse that you had arrived. That wasn't until a month after your appearance, so you can understand that Daddy was rather worried.
>
> From what Mommie tells me and Ethel [Kennedy's mother-in-law] (I'm sure you'll be calling her Ethel before long and loving her too) and from the pictures I've had, you must be a very lovely little girl. Daddy can never tell you how anxious he is to see you. He loves you very, very much.
>
> I'm sure that even at this early date you've already recognized what a perfect mother you have—and you're quite right, 'cause she is. Paulie and Joanie and I love her very much and you do too, only it will be a while before you know it. Each day you're with her will teach you something new about her—something new to love. That's the way it has been with me, so it will be with you.
>
> This has been a difficult war for many of us—more for some than for others. From little more than nothing to the last breath of life have been given—that's a wide variance but always, Ruthie, the willingness to give everything was about the same.
>
> Though we don't like to think of it and though it isn't very possible, there's always a chance that you'll never know your Daddy—accidents happen so easily at times. I don't want to worry your pretty little head or Mommie's either, but I just want you to know that anything worthwhile that I've done was done because I love you and Mommie and Paulie and Joanie, and because I want you to go on having the chances I've had—to go on living in such a wonderful country such as ours is. I promise you, Ruthie, that it is just that, so believe me until you have a chance to know it through yourself.

I hope you've had a happy birthday and I pray that before you're much older I'll be with you. Daddy sends all his love to you (and tell Mommie I love her more than ever).

Lovingly,
Daddy

Tuesday, July 25, 1944

Wrote letters all morning and had a good swim this afternoon. One of our enlisted men was drowned yesterday in another part of the beach. Played a double-header ball game this evening with the 11th Evac. Got word, too, that we're going into a staging area with the division tomorrow. We'll be stripped of everything in our new area so life won't be so good. I think our days in Italy are very few. The end of the war is so near, yet so much lies ahead of us. I pray to God that I'll come out of this OK.

Wednesday, July 26, 1944

Tore down this morning and then had to wait 'til this afternoon for moving orders. We only had 15 miles to move but it was over the coast road—dusty and bumpy—toward Naples. We're set up in an apple and pear orchard and in a pretty comfortable spot. No tents so it'll be too bad if it rains. Radio working fine so we had music and news all evening. Very hot and quite dusty, however, and of course there's no way to shower or take a bath. We'll be here a few days so we're all going to hightail it into Naples tomorrow and stay for a few days.

Thursday, July 27, 1944

Everybody into Naples right after breakfast and went out to 21st General and made rounds. Cases coming back in pretty good shape. Saw two of our bilateral amputations all healed and ready for the States. Had dinner out there, then back to the Red Cross—later up to Allied Orange Club—had dinner and drinks there, then home by 12:00 to our apple orchard.

Saturday, July 29, 1944

Packed again today—I've increased my bedding roll to quite a package but it's comfortable, to say the least. Went to Mass at 4 p.m. over in the 111th Clearing area. Father Murphy back here for dinner—had fried chicken and it was good. Drove the truck over to the 36th Division area to a movie—*Once upon a Time*—a silly story but quite entertaining.

Heard all sorts of rumors today. M. [Madding] says we're hitting in nine places—a big movement, airborne troops, et al. I'm beginning to believe that I'm not gonna enjoy this too much.

Sunday, July 30, 1944

Mass this morning over at the 11th Evac. The colonel has them tied down and they're wild. Went to town on the thumb this morning and it took me a couple hours to go 14 miles. Had a fine dinner with Major Townsend and then spent the night there with him at the 118th Station. The harbor looked awfully full to me. Of course I was quizzed by him and some of his friends and was held in awe—"Here's a D-day soldier"—so to speak. I wish people would stop talking about it. I'd feel a lot better.

Wednesday, August 2, 1944

Mail broke the monotony of this day—did all right but got only one letter from Marion. Got a package from M. [Marion] with a couple cans of beer in it which I had this evening—mighty good. Still just sitting and waiting. Feel this weekend will see the end of it and we'll get out of here. Looking over some maps today and I'm not too sure now that we're going to France—it may well be Yugoslavia. It is the shortest way into Berlin from here, and with the Russians driving toward Krakow we'd pinch off a lot in the Balkan states.

Thursday, August 3, 1944

Assembled with the 36th Division officers this afternoon to hear Major General Truscott deliver a charge to them (us) on the coming operation. Three divisions abreast against the heaviest defended coastline that we've yet attempted to breach (what're they doing to me?)—great navy and air support promised—"You've done great work in the past—Salerno, Cassino, Anzio—and now this, your last job, will be your greatest."

It's hard to believe that in a little while many of the group I stood behind will be dead or severely wounded, but it will happen. God damn this war!

Tuesday, August 8, 1944

In town right after breakfast—this was our last day, supposedly—caught a ride right to the Red Cross door (I'm still bumming). Breakfast and a shower—the Red Cross routine. Harbor loaded with ships and the O.D.s seen in town are few and far between. Had seven scoops of ice cream at the Red Cross at 7 p.m., then home. Got six letters from Marion but too dark to answer them. Word we're moving to a new area in the morning. From there to the boats the next day.

Wednesday, August 9, 1944

Restricted this morning and for once all our group was in the area. This is really a sight—troops scattered all over the place—dust a foot thick—nobody has anything except the stuff he can carry. My bedding roll is a little too heavy but tonight this air mattress feels pretty good and it's worth the effort. It's really down-to-earth living and is endurable only because you know it isn't for long—the poor infantry lives like this all the time, and frequently dies in it. They've been marching by all evening into the field next to us—heavy packs and a heavier rifle. My lot isn't too bad, I guess.

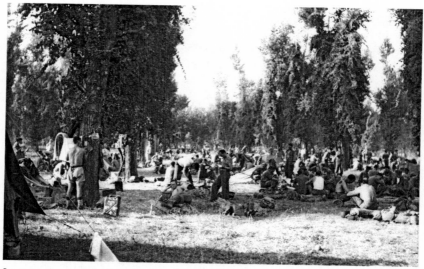

Last staging area before the invasion of southern France.

Thursday, August 10, 1944

Aboard the U.S.N. transport *General George O. Squier*

Had a poor night last night—the British right behind us drank scotch 'til all hours. Up at dawn to start a long wait 'til noon. Had cold meat and beans for breakfast. Large truck convoy to Naples and the docks—greeted there at 1:00 by the Red Cross with doughnuts and lemonade (pretty good). Ship is a new navy transport (2,500 troops) and the accommodations excellent, much to our surprise. Room for 18 but only 10 of us in it. Had a saltwater bath (hot and filthy dirty when we boarded), then later had an excellent dinner. (Another real surprise—we expected C rations.) I'm certain where we're going but we'll see—and it won't take long to get there.

Friday, August 11, 1944
On ship—

Pulled away from the harbor of Naples and sailed across the bay to Castelammare, where we're lying at anchor with other transports and L.S.T.s, most of them combat loaded.

Weather still hot but cloudy—rained hard last night. Meals still excellent and ship more comfortable than anyone expected. (They sell ice cream on board here that is excellent and there seems to be plenty of it.) (The navy lives right!) Still lots of speculation as per usual as to where we're going. I got a job assigned to me—a watch from 4 a.m. to 8 a.m.

Saturday, August 12, 1944
On ship

Still just off Castelammare sitting in a blazing hot sun and minding the heat more all the time. Up at 4 a.m. to sit out watch from then 'til 8 a.m.—a long four hours in a dark hatch filled with sweating soldiers. Fortunate your sense of smell tires after a time and you smell nothing. Eating two meals a day with sandwich at noon, and the food continues excellent. Reading—on my bunk, on deck, a saltwater shower, ice cream, more speculation—signs!! The L.S.T.s pulled out this evening—a sign we may go tonight or early tomorrow. This waiting is difficult, particularly for something that might be disastrous.

Sunday, August 13, 1944
At sea

Up for my watch at 4 a.m. to find us still at anchor. My watch interrupts my sleep no end. To Mass and Communion at 9 a.m. Pulled anchor and sailed at 1300 hours—all the transports that were around us plus a few line ships. Speed pretty good—must be 18 knots—wasn't long before we were at sea. Four hours out all C.O.s were briefed on the mission, but we've not been enlightened as yet. Our general guess was right. Got my money back in francs—13 500-franc notes. A Grumman Wildcat zoomed past us—there are many carriers in the vicinity, so the story goes. But you can hear anything you want on the ship.

Monday, August 14, 1944

At sea—on eve of D-day.

What I feel—the million things that are running thru my mind would more than fill this page. What happens tomorrow can be so disastrous in so many ways. I hope and pray that all goes well.

The day has been very quiet. More ships have joined us—battlewagons among them, other transports, but we can see only a small part of the task force. There's no great excitement among the men though they know as well as anyone that tomorrow may be their end. The morale is good and most everyone feels that only success will be ours. I'm sure it will but I'm not sure of the price.

[The invasion of southern France, Operation Dragoon, was originally intended to coincide with Overlord, but a shortage of landing craft delayed it for more than two months. In addition, Churchill resisted the entire concept on the grounds that it would sap the strength of the forces in Italy. The idea that Italy provided a route for an invasion of Germany from the south was suspect at the time, and indeed in retrospect, appears almost ludicrous. The difficulties of attacking and overcoming entrenched German defensive positions were manifest in Italy; they would have been magnified exponentially in the Alps.

Under the overall command of General Alexander Patch, leader of the Seventh Army, the American VI Corps, consisting of the Forty-Fifth, Thirty-Sixth, and Third divisions and supported by the French II Corps, landed between Cannes and Toulon against light resistance on August 15. Opposing the landing was German Army Group G, commanded by General Johannes Blaskowitz. In the face of superior Allied strength, and commanding an army that had been stripped of much of its equipment and many of its first-line troops, Blaskowitz had no choice but to withdraw. This resulted in a rapid Allied advance up the valley of the Rhone.

To illustrate the speed of the Allies' advance—and to contrast it with the stagnation of the war in Italy—between October 5, 1943, and March 3, 1944, in Italy, GST 6 moved seven times; between August 15, 1944, and January 7, 1945, in France—in roughly the same amount of time— GST 6/26 set up in twenty-six separate locations in their efforts to keep up with the front.

By September 11—less than a month after coming ashore—advance units of the Seventh Army met Patton's Third Army north of Dijon; the Allied forces now stood ready to turn east and into Germany itself.]

Tuesday, August 15, 1944

Le Dramont Plage on the Riviera

Things started to happen at 5:30 this morning while I was on my watch. Naval guns throwing salvo after salvo into the beach area. At 7 it stopped, and heavy bombers in waves of 36 each then came out of the southwest and hit the beach area. Just before the first assault wave went in to land at 8:00, ships mounting hundreds of rockets "peppered" the beach. We landed at H 10 riding from our transport 15 miles out on an L.C.I. Uneventful ride in—landed on green beach. Things seemed a bit confused—100 prisoners waiting on the beach to be taken out to a ship. They were shelling the beach occasionally so we got out of there (loaded down) and found a bivouac area for the night on the side of a hill overlooking this little town. At 9 p.m., just at dusk, a Jerry plane came in from the east and when it was still 1,000 yards from the beach it released a robot radio-controlled bomb which flew just ahead of the plane and then gracefully slid downward and hit an L.S.T. square on the bridge. Flames and a terrific explosion and the L.S.T. burned and exploded all night. Four Long Toms were on it plus lots of ammunition.

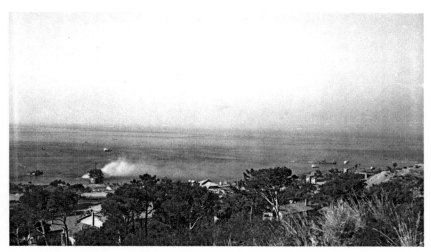

Burning LST on Green Beach

No other ships lost. There were three other beaches but news from there is scarce tonight. 155s are just below us and are firing over us—the noise is terrible—that plus the ack-ack would wake the dead. We're right in the middle of it too and the flak falls too close. I've got my bed laid out in a ditch with a door lying crossways over my head. Here's where an air mattress comes in mighty handy.

I've landed on D-day and I'm all in one piece, thank God. Things seem to be going well although they're only six miles from the water as yet. There was little resistance here, and with the way the Normandy front is going I think we'll meet little.

Wednesday, August 16, 1944

In a villa on the French Riviera just east of San Raphael. Had a good night in spite of the noise, et al. Explored the countryside this morning, and this place looks like a war hit it all of a sudden. I can see that it was a beautiful place in peacetime—villas all overlooking the sea—small coves that seem to be separate little lakes hidden from everything, war included. Saw Jerry pillboxes dotting the hill that naval shells blasted out of existence.

The L.S.T. still burning. Many prisoners in the 36 Division P.O.W. enclosures. Not looking too happy.

Progress is good. The 155s have moved up some and we have a house to sleep in. Tomorrow we're setting up six miles from here on a golf course.

Thursday, August 17, 1944

One mile south of Le Muy

Had another robot bomb thrown at the beach last night just after sunset. We could hear it roaring, getting closer all the time, and everyone dove for the floor—it hit the water and exploded. A 155 is just outside our yard and it fired a mission (15 rounds), almost making me deaf. We waited around all day to move and finally left at 3:00 in a 6 x 6—passed thru San Raphael, Frejus. French flags flying from every house—people all in a holiday mood waving to us.

More prisoners coming in; walking, in trucks, and all seem not too unhappy. Glider traps covered the fields hereabout—poles with barbed wire strung between them. We set up just a mile south of Le Muy. 11th Evac next door.

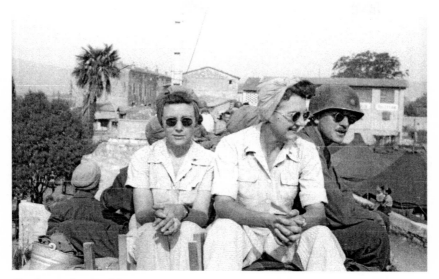

On the road to Le Muy

Friday, August 18, 1944

Draguignan, France

Moved here this afternoon and set up immediately—patients already waiting. Clean-looking town and people much improved. The countryside is pretty. We passed a couple fields on the way here that had hundreds of broken-up gliders in them. Jerry had lots of glider traps around.

Jerry had cleared out of here yesterday, so you see even the medics are close on his heels. There's a building right behind us that a shell hit this morning—it's still burning and fires are burning on the hill just ahead of us. Did one Jerry belly this evening.

Saturday, August 19, 1944

Patients have been nil all day. I guess nobody is getting seriously wounded. The advance is still rapid and the news from Normandy is excellent—the Jerry 7th Army is in rout. Went into Draguignan this morning to look around. No war damage worth mentioning—people all very cordial and seem honestly pleased that we are here. One fellow who could talk English said that the Germans were correct but not nice—the Americans are nice. Bought some perfume for Marion and a French book for Paulie. They have beer here in this town but in no way does it resemble our beer. Hospital is moving in a.m. but we're staying behind as a holding company.

Sunday, August 20, 1944

Again we're miles behind the front. There's been no resistance of any great amount and the 36th Division is going ahead rapidly. We're going to move again tomorrow about 100 miles—if this keeps up it won't be long before we're nearing Paris. Toulon and Marseilles, however, haven't fallen as yet. Went to Mass over at the clearing station (Father Murphy).

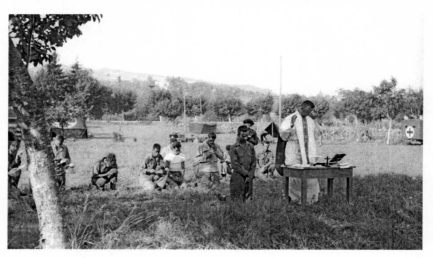

Mass in the field

Charlie Westerfield [Charles W. Westerfield, anesthetist] and I took a walk up the side hill back of the town to get some figs and in doing so we met a French family who told us of conditions hereabout—food is a real problem—eggs are 30¢ apiece, no flour or meat. They raise a few rabbits and eat them occasionally.

Monday, August 21, 1944

Tore down right after breakfast and all eight teams and equipment mounted three trucks with trailers and we were off. A sight hard to imagine so I took a picture of it.

We traveled over 100 miles through some beautiful country, quite mountainous 'cause we're just in the foothills of the French Alps. Unlike Italy, the countryside and the people that line the road as you go by

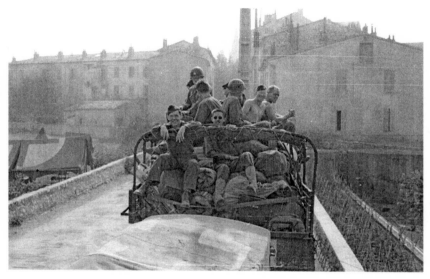

Overloaded truck and trailer on the road to Volonne

appear clean. I never heard such enthusiastic cheering and clapping—I believe they are very sincere. Went north to Castellans, Digne, then west to Volonne on the Durance River (the headwaters of the Rhone). Tonight the line is 50 kilometers ahead of us and is moving fast. Radio news from Normandy is excellent. We're already across the Seine River in one place.

Tuesday, August 22, 1944

This war is moving much too fast for the Medical Department. Finally had to take the two platoons and form a half an evac hospital—got in 80 patients today, of which only a few were casualties. We're again about 100 miles behind things but we're moving again tomorrow. I drove back to Digne this morning with Father Murphy. I there met the bishop of Digne. F.M. tried to talk to him in Latin but the good bishop's Latin is a little weak. Stopped in a Jerry hospital and talked with one of the medical officers. They seemed not at all unhappy about what was happening. On our way back here we saw some Maquis[3] bringing in five Jerry prisoners—that was at least 50 miles behind our hospital site.

Wednesday, August 23, 1944

Borsuk's platoon has moved on ahead a little, over 100 miles, so we're moving up there in shifts. We have been packed and all ready to go all day but the trucks didn't get back 'til after dark so we're staying here overnight. These roads are dangerous—many curves and lots of cliffs. Radio announced the fall of Paris to the F.F.I.[4] today. Talked to a Maquis here this afternoon. He spoke fair English. The gun he had and the hand grenades were American. They were dropped by parachute over two years ago. Supplies have continued to fall in that way ever since.

Thursday, August 24, 1944

Left this morning after breakfast—two trucks loaded to the hilt plus one truck to ride in. Went thru beautiful country on the way—winding mountain roads, high peaks, and beautiful deep green valleys. Stopped at the 36 Division A.P.O. on the way and mailed several letters to Marion. First mail we've had go out. Went to Serres, then to Die, and finally to our area near Crest. Again we were enthusiastically welcomed by the French along the way. Had a bath in a little creek just below us—cool, clear water—Kaplan and I got caught in the nude by a French gal—she smiled, waved, and ran away. Having fairly heavy casualties and we're getting them all here. Three tables going all the time.

Friday, August 25, 1944

Walked up to Crest this afternoon and looked around. Nice little town and people very friendly. Had a glass of vin blanc in the Cafe des Alpes. They invited us for dinner tomorrow. As we were leaving, some excited townsfolk rushed up to us and asked if the Germans were coming. Just at that moment Father Murphy came flying back from division C.P. in his jeep with the news that the 11th Panzer Division was coming down the road toward Crest. We can hear machine-gun and small-arms fire tonight and large shells are hitting on the hillside behind us—much too close. It seems we have Jerry on all three sides of us—north, west, and south.

Saturday, August 26, 1944

An exciting day with an even more exciting night in the offing. It seems we're virtually surrounded, with the only road out to the east under shell fire and observation by the Germans. All last night heavy shells hit around us and mighty close too. More than once I hit the dirt and hugged the earth with a fierce love. We had the night shift again so we were up practically all night. This morning all patients that could possibly be moved were evacuated. The nurses have been moved to a hill behind us and there have been dug in. G. and I have a very comfortable foxhole in our tent. There's a road running north thru Crest over which a Jerry panzer division is trying to move north. We hold Crest (two kilometers from here)—so tonight may be a thriller—or a dud. Not exciting, but I prefer the latter.

Sunday, August 27, 1944

Worked all last night and when we went off this morning shock was still full. As far as any trouble with Jerry goes, we had none. A correspondent in here today said the division turned up the Rhone valley and got away only because we had too little here to hold them. Patients coming in—and there were plenty of them—said that Jerry paid a pretty good price to get away. The hospital suffered none—went on full blast, as per usual. Me 109s were over at treetop level strafing the road just below us and we got in a couple drivers they hit. It's been boiling hot here all day and I haven't slept a wink. But we go back on at 12 tonight.

Monday, August 28, 1944

We had a complete night's sleep though we were on second call. Had one case today but it was a beauty. A fellow in a tank had a Jerry 88 explode so close to his face that it singed his hair. His whole face from his eyes down is missing. Right arm amputated, too, at the shoulder, plus a thousand other wounds. Better that he should die.

Two Jerry planes over today strafing the road below us. Seeing them quite frequently now.

Tuesday, August 29, 1944

We had a short shift but I don't believe I could have taken anymore. We worked constantly from 8 this morning to 6 tonight—did four real major cases. One a 15-year-old French kid. He died this evening. The shock ward is still full but we're off now. Charlie W. and I went down to the

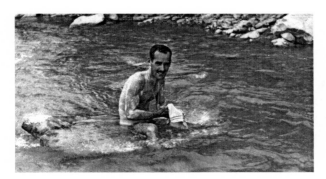

Charlie Westerfield
near Crest, France

creek and had a bath, then walked down the road to our French friends. They cooked a chicken for us, made a salad, and brought out some wine, and we ate and talked (Charlie did the talking) for a couple hours. I couldn't keep my eyes open any longer so we went home. They are happy no end that the Americans are here and don't hesitate to show it.

Wednesday, August 30, 1944

Feeling sick to my stomach—have all day. Guess our French meal of last night didn't agree with me.

Work has suddenly shut down here—didn't have a single case all day. P.O.W.s are not being sent over from the clearing station—conserving our supplies for our own boys—which is right.

Down to the creek for a bath—I have a hell of a time hanging onto the soap in that rushing water and as a result I've lost almost all I have.

News tonight says statement by minister of propaganda in Germany suggests to German people that the war is lost. I hope they do something about it now and quit.

Friday, September 1, 1944

Last of the clearing station moved out this afternoon—ahead of us 50 miles. We may move tomorrow. Charlie W. & I walked into Crest today— had lunch with a French family that we ran across in trying to buy some berets. Had a good meal, too—eggs, potatoes, tomatoes, beans, melon, and pear. Back for a swim in the creek—then found mail—first since we arrived in France and it was more than welcome.

Saturday, September 2, 1944

Crest, Chabeuil, Romans, Baurepaire, Cour et buis, Diemoz (south of Heyrieux)

Red Walker rudely awakened us at 5:30 with the news we were to move over a 100 miles to a spot just south of Lyons. Mad rush as usual— stuff piled high on the trucks in 2nd Aux fashion and off—10 minutes out of Crest we got caught in rain and it rained for the entire trip. No cover—not even a field jacket—so we got soaked thru to the skin and stayed that way for hours. We scared up some blankets but they soon were wet. Moved into our new area in a pouring rain and set up in a field of mud. Our tent leaks like a sieve so I've got a pup tent over my bed. The 36th Division is lining up to take Lyons, but this rain will hold them up. They're seven miles ahead of us tonight.

Sunday, September 3, 1944

The rains let up as soon as they came, and everything is drying today. Beautiful country around here—reminds me much of Groton. Mass at the clearing station at 11—weather cold enough for a combat jacket. The French for miles around are milling through here curious to see how the Americans live. Dressed in their finest and looking quite nice, too, they were here by the hundreds. Took some pictures of some kids that were cute as the devil. Did one case here and that not a battle casualty. The line is 35 miles above Lyons tonight.

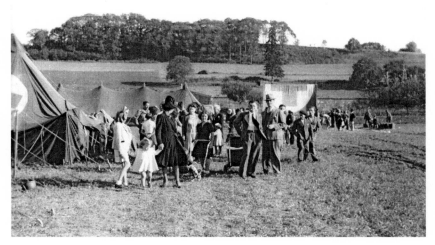

French visitors

Monday, September 4, 1944

Quite a day in Lyons. Got news at 8 this morning that we were going to move up 65 miles this evening, so we decided we'd see Lyons in the meantime, not knowing its exact status. Hitched in and made good time—about 17 miles from here. Lyons is a big city—800,000 population—and seems to be quite modern. The Saone River joins the Rhone in the center of the city, and it was at the immediate vicinity of the rivers that most of the action in Lyons took place. The Germans blew all bridges before they left Saturday night and knocked everything down except the Woodrow Wilson Bridge over the Rhone and one suspension bridge over the Saone.

As we entered the downtown section we were just in time to see a group of F.F.I. men rounding up two collaborators. Followed by a large crowd, which we joined, they carried the two poor guys upside down into a building and beat the devil out of them. We, like dumb clucks, followed them in and saw it all. Went on downtown then, getting big waves, hellos, and much greeting from all sides. Stores were all closed but so far there was little destruction. By this time we had picked up three French boys (18 or so) that spoke English and they proceeded to take us over the Rhone. We later crossed over the Saone into the part of the city not yet quite settled. Got into a little restaurant for lunch and when they discovered we were Americans they couldn't do enough for us. A pretty French girl insisted on kissing us all—both-cheek style. Had wine, meat, bread, and Roquefort cheese. As we came out of the place—along the Saone shots rang out and machine guns began to rattle. All of a sudden we found ourselves in the middle of a street fight between the collaborators and the F.F.I. We crouched behind the wall for over half an hour with an occasional "zing" from bullets whizzing overhead. We dashed across the bridge and thru some back streets over to the Rhone, where there was more firing. They had some collaborators pinned in the tower of a hospital on the Rhone, and they were in the process of smoking them out.

Took lots of pictures of this. Finally got home to find we were moving in the a.m. Norris Frank's tent burned down while we were at supper.

Tuesday, September 5, 1944

Up at 5:30 to get an early start, but as usual we hurried to wait. Finally away at 8 a.m. in a weapons carrier. All but two teams staying behind to wait for transportation. Again riding thru beautiful country. Crossed the Rhone and the Ain. Clever bridge put up across the Rhone.

Bridge out at Pont d'Ain. They had a good fight there. Buildings burned out, etc. Thru Bourg to Attignat and stayed for night. Situation all bawled up as usual. Back into Bourg to see the town—had dinner in the Grande Hotel.

Wednesday, September 6, 1944

Off again in the a.m. was just a little bit wrong. It's now 7 p.m. and we're still sitting waiting for transportation. Went in Bonry and stayed 'til 3:30. Had lunch at the Europa Hotel—another excellent meal. General Patch, 7th Army commander, ate at the next table to us. This afternoon I saw Les Poulets[5] being herded into a large van along one of the main streets in

Bonry—a large crowd pushed and crowded around cheering and jeering. Their heads were shaved and swastikas were painted on their foreheads in lipstick. Quite a sight.

Thursday, September 7, 1944

The trucks came for us at midnight. I was just getting asleep when I had to get up and pack. Rode most of the night in a command car to our new area 63 miles north of Bourg, three kilometers south of Poligny. It was a beautiful night all the way even as we unloaded in the new area, but just as soon as we had set up our cots and had gotten in, it started to pour and in a very few minutes we were soaked. They immediately set up a ward tent but the damage had already been done. Spent most of today trying to get dry. Went into Poligny and had an excellent meal—it's almost a Swiss town—sort of Alpine architecture. People not enthusiastic but awfully bitter toward the Germans. Talked to one woman whose brother they shot the past week. A man told us of one they cut hands off with a buzz saw. We hear such stories constantly.

Friday, September 8, 1944

Got a room in 76 Hotel Paris last night—our bedding was still wet. A nice clean little hotel with good beds but convoys went by all night (it's sheep you count, not convoys).

Our team was sent to Chalon this morning by 7th Army surgeon to see an American officer who had been operated on by a French civilian surgeon. We took our instruments and blood but found the patient doing well—so we saw Chalon. No Americans there at all. Had a fine dinner—roast beef. Heard more stories of German atrocities. The French say there is no word to describe the Germans—savage doesn't half say it, they claim. Traded two packs of cigs for a bottle of Evening in Paris. Back here to find the clearing station gone, but we're staying until tomorrow.

Saturday, September 9, 1944

Cold as the very devil at night and during the day when the clouds hide the sun. Winter comes closer as we go north. We moved this afternoon to Lavans Guinney, some 20 miles. Came thru Arbois, the home of Louis Pasteur. Saw his home and the little building where he did his work. Were about 25 kilometers from Besancon. We're bivouacked here and will probably move on in the morning. This present site is very pretty—we're on a knoll which overlooks several valleys and from here you can see three little villages. France is really beautiful.

Monday, September 11, 1944

Trucks arrived for us early this a.m. and took first load, but it was afternoon by the time they got us. Moved about 45 miles—near Fretigney. When we got here the line was 17 miles north of us, but now they say they're advancing rapidly again. Hospital was set up expecting some casualties, but now it looks like we'll get none. On the way up here we passed a large number of Jerry prisoners—some of them were digging graves to bury some of their own dead that were piled nearby.

Tuesday, September 12, 1944

Rooted out of bed at 4 a.m. this morning and did a couple cases. Vesoul about 18 miles from here is the objective. Looks like we'll be busy here for a while. I've been feeling sick at my stomach all day and my gut is griping terribly. Been quite a bit of it in the outfit. Red Walker, head of this platoon, got his promotion to major today and this evening he had us all in for drinks.

First news of Americans entering Germany came thru B.B.C. today. Maybe the end won't be far off. Letter from Marion—told of Leo Klauberg's [an acquaintance of the Kennedys] death in Normandy.

Wednesday, September 13, 1944

Worked until 5 a.m. so tonight I'm about bushed. Clearing station moved out today so I guess our work here will be short lived.

Raining all day and the tent has leaked continually. I've got my pup tent set up over my bed so I'm fairly dry. At night when you look up at the tent roof it looks like the Hayden Planetarium.

Thursday, September 14, 1944

Started in at noon today and just finished up—1 a.m.—had a nephrectomy, among other things. We're actually running a P.O.W. hospital. We chase them like hell—shoot hell out of them—and then work like hell to keep them alive—for what?

Colonel Forsee and Major Sullivan blew in today—mail came at same time and I got a pretty good deal, but as per usual after reading it I feel more lonesome than ever. Nothing new from headquarters.

Friday, September 15, 1944

Worked until 3 this morning—mostly Jerries. Rain cleared and sun came out, drying everything rapidly. Got orders to move at 2 p.m. and by 3 we

were on the road—moved up 10 miles beyond Vesuol on the road to Luxe-
uil. A very pretty flat but low area. If it rains we'll be inundated—only three
teams here so we'll work 24-hour shifts (too much). Corps surgeon warned
us that there are isolated units of Jerries behind us that we must be careful
of at night. They've been trying to get away in stolen American vehicles.

Saturday, September 16, 1944

Got a case in at 11:00 and worked 'til 2 this morning—in bed by 3 a.m.
Worked practically all day on one case—a French woman (30 years
old)—who rode over a land mine on a bicycle. Bilateral amputation
through the thighs plus a million other wounds [case 170]. Her husband
came in with her and it was a pitiful sight to watch him saying good-bye
as he left the O.R.

> Case 170. Diagnosis 1) Amp. incomplete, traumatic, rt. lower
> leg 2) F.C.C. fib & tib, rt. & left, sv.) Wds. pen & perf multiple
> abd. chest walls 4) Wds pen & perf multiple both hands, fore-
> arms, and arms 5) F.C.C. metacarpal rt. 5th 6) Blindness incom-
> plete, eye, left 7) Wds pen & perf multiple face.

This evening a Jerry a chest wound comes in, still boasting that Hitler is the great man and that Germany will win the war—and we work
to save his life.

Sunday, September 17, 1944

Woke up this morning to find the entire area under 10 inches of water—
no matter where you looked you saw just water. The one time our tent
didn't leak, the water came up through the floor. Things were so miserable that we actually could do nothing but laugh at our predicament. Was
told division put us there—they blamed it on corps. Corps came back at
division and division came back at the C.O. of the hospital (army buck
passing). We had to move in all that rain and water a quarter of a mile
away. We're up on a hill tonight and fairly dry, but it will be weeks before
my shoes dry out.

Monday, September 18, 1944

Went into Luxueil this morning—noted for its natural hot springs around
which baths have been built. It was also the home of the Escadrille Lafayette in World War I. Germans left Friday night.

We met a French doctor and his family who invited us in to dinner—had a delicious five-course meal. Wine, champagne, and cognac. He even had real coffee. They talked English and were extremely interesting. Another example of the warmth with which the French welcomed the Americans—not so with the English.

Tuesday, September 19, 1944

Rain all day but slowly—no patients coming in 'cause the 36th is resting two days (for clean dry clothes and shoes and a few hot meals). We're moving again tomorrow so I hope the rain stops for a while. I'm afraid now that the weather is gonna prolong this thing and it won't end as quickly as the newspapers would have you believe. Gordon and Kaplan went over to Lure this morning, but the fighting was a little too close. It was the center of the American medical setup in World War I.

Wednesday, September 20, 1944

Into Luxueil to 11th Field headquarters for a hot shower. Traffic north is extremely heavy. Back, did laundry and then just waited around 'til dark to move. For no good reason at all we wait all day to hurry up and move at night. 36 Division Q.M. (Hell Drivers, they call themselves) moved us, and I really understand how they got their name—blackout driving, plunging ahead into what looked like complete blackness. How he ever saw the road is a mystery to me—but he did. We're just south of Plombieres and only about six miles short of the Moselle River. It seems we're piling up stuff here to drive east sharply toward Belfort.

Thursday, September 21, 1944

Hospital was all set up and ready for patients at 4 a.m. this morning. That's pretty good for pitching in complete darkness.

We've been on all day and as per usual when we're on we're always busy. The attempt to cross the Moselle last night wasn't exactly a success. If we're this busy you can be sure the total casualties are high.

It's 2 a.m.—to bed.

Friday, September 22, 1944

Walked into Plombieres this morning about a mile and a half north of here. Pretty little town with natural warm springs and so there are numerous elaborate *bains* [baths]. Had a fair lunch—rabbit. Came back to find lots of work, which will keep us going all night. Operated on Charles Dorish from Wilkes Barre this evening.

Mail came in this afternoon and as always it makes me more lonesome than ever. My whole family and Marion's are agreed that Paulie, Joanie, and Ruthie are the most beautiful children they've ever seen, and the smartest.

Saturday, September 23, 1944

Didn't finish work 'til breakfast time this morning. I slept until 11 but had to get up then to do post-op care. Raining cats and dogs all night and all day but we're dry. The ward is full, so we're evacuating all possible to 9th Evac, which is unusually close: three miles. Getting almost nothing but small-arms injuries now—most unusual.

Clearing station supposed to move tomorrow so a platoon will follow them. Looks like we're going to hold and I welcome a chance to sit. It's 7:30 only but I can't keep my eyes open any longer.

Sunday, September 24, 1944

Still raining. The sun appears each evening at just about dusk and gives brief promise of a nice day to come. But it turns out to be only a promise and we get the usual rain. To Mass at the clearing station in a tent full of mud, but Mass just the same. We're on all day but most everything is going to the 9th Evac. We're closed for moving tomorrow.

The airborne army is still out on a limb in Holland. I wonder if that's gonna be another Anzio.

Monday, September 25, 1944

Still raining and it's bitter cold. I almost froze last night. Red's platoon moved up ahead of us and all our teams but us. We're holding what's left. After the others left we got in four cases which have kept us busy all day (and which will keep us here a few days longer). I get fed up very easily, I guess, but all this rain and cold—this lousy food and no mail puts me down and sits on me. I want so badly to go home to my family—and I feel so sure that it's still gonna be a long way off.

Wednesday, September 27, 1944

The airborne were pulled back over the Rhine from Arnhem. From all accounts they've had a wicked stand.

Still raining here but each day progress is being reported on the 7th Army front, but the overall picture has slowed to almost a standstill. The general thought here is that it will last 'til next spring, and I believe that's a good guess. A few weeks ago I thought it would be all over by Xmas, but now I'm sure that that's too optimistic a hope.

Have a Jerry stove in our tent and it's a devil to keep going—it burns paper nicely but that's about all.

Monday, October 2, 1944

Got rid of all our patients this morning and moved right after lunch to Eloyes—about 17 miles north toward Epinal. Fighting is four miles off to the east near a town named Tendon. The river is just a few hundred yards down in front of us. Beyond that are some low hills which separate us from the battle. We're right in the middle of the artillery and it promises to be rather noisy. Some Jerry shells have fallen awfully close to the hospital. For once we're set up in a French day nursery and the living is fine—a floor and a roof. The hospital itself is still in tents.

Tuesday, October 3, 1944

Went on call this morning at 8 and we've had a busy day. It seems that as soon as we hit a place they always get busy. Did five cases and they were all big ones. Had some Jerry planes strafing the road here at noon—three of them. Some of our own shells fell and exploded just beyond the hospital but no one was injured. About a mile down the road one of them was shot down (good!).

There are over 30 patients in the hospital—a large number for non-transportable cases—and they're all sick. There are two cute little French kids, four and five years old, both with belly wounds.

Wednesday, October 4, 1944

Not on call 'til midnight but nothing's coming in so maybe we'll work the night shift in bed. Sully down today but no mail with him. Hospital now at Epinal—north of us. Gordon had a war correspondent in tow here today—a Mr. Cook of *Newsweek*. He's gonna do a story on auxiliary surgical teams.

Had a movie at headquarters today—wasn't any good but if strength comes from length, it had it. Patients of yesterday doing OK—my bladder case seems to be all right.

Eloyes is just a little town, a main street and nothing more. A large cotton mill supports the town and everybody seems to have worked there before the war. Today we took a walk over there just to see it—just across the Moselle. Some F.F.I. were leading a middle-aged woman and her three small children down to the town hall. We and some other officers were let in to her trial—an informal affair at which she was hardly represented. Accused of rather intimate relations with Jerry, she was convicted and immediately the sentence was carried out—her head was promptly shaved. The oldest boy (14) knew the charge and cried bitterly, hiding his face in his hands—but he stood by his mother. Once turned loose, she and her brood paraded home, receiving from all sides the jeers of her town—the cheers of the G.I.s that walked the street. We went home then with our hair but a little ashamed.

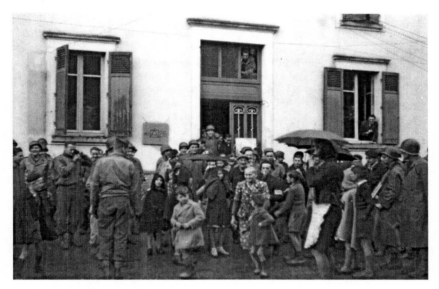

Newly shaven Poulet in Éloyes

Thursday, October 5, 1944

Got thru the night without a call but got a nice case this noon—a laceration of the inferior vena cava just after it went into the liver. We left two long clamps on the thing and retired gracefully. The fellow's still kicking today but I fear that it won't be for long [case 194].

> Case 194. Diagnosis: S.F. wds. multiple pen thorax right sv; abdomen, rt. sv; buttocks rt. sv.; ankle, rt sv. F.B. (small) in ankle joint. Patient expired 10-10-44 at 0009 hrs.

Raining and cold here—more artillery than usual. The 3rd Division is south and a little west of us, firing sort of northeast —their shells fly over like empty freight cars.

Movie tonight at 11th headquarters—not bad at all.

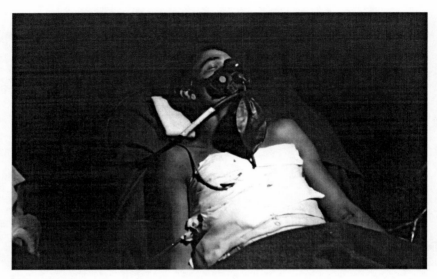

Case 194

Friday, October 6, 1944

Work has definitely slowed up. The weather has improved so I should think they'd try to make some kind of a drive, but no.

Had an inspection today by Major General Kenner, surgeon to SHAEF [Supreme Headquarters Allied Expeditionary Force].[6] (He was a colonel when we came into Casablanca.) He asked some awfully stupid questions for a guy who's supposed to be the boss of all medical installations.

Sunday, October 8, 1944

Beautiful sunny day. 11:00 o'clock Mass at the clearing station. Father Murphy is being transferred to the 143rd Infantry Regiment soon, so we'll be without a priest here at the clearing station. It's been good having Father Murphy around and I'll miss him when he goes.

Very little work coming in—only casualties are those caused by Jerry's mortar—which is deadly, they say. There's no progress here at all. The artillery is still in our front yard.

Monday, October 9, 1944

More rain, but living in a building and having a little heat makes living in the rain not too bad. Had a distinguished visitor in this region today.

General [George Catlett] Marshal [Jr.]—chief of staff. Somebody who was at division C.P. said there was a grand total of 26 stars around. I hope they thought up something good to do around here, 'cause to my untrained eye it looks like they're getting nowhere fast.

Heard the final game of the World Series tonight—my Browns lost!

Tuesday, October 10, 1944

Raining again but fairly warm. On since last midnight but we only worked the day part of our shift. Had two chest cases. We're beginning to see pulmonary complications now similar to those we experienced last winter in Italy. They all seem to have a tracheo bronchitis when they come in.

Wednesday, October 11, 1944

On the all-afternoon and night-'til-morning shift but so far no business. Two cases in but Chunn [Charles F. Chunn, general surgeon]—the eager beaver—is doing them. Miss Hall had a party tonight—her first anniversary working. They had some pretty good food but I had no drinks because of being on call. A little mail came in but only newspapers for me. For some reason or other I feel particularly low tonight. There's no sign here that this war is gonna be over this year and I just can't bear to think of not getting home 'til next summer—but that's what it's gonna be.

Saturday, October 14, 1944

Raining all day but now it's an accepted thing and doesn't seem to interrupt proceedings very much. Things very quiet as far as work is con-

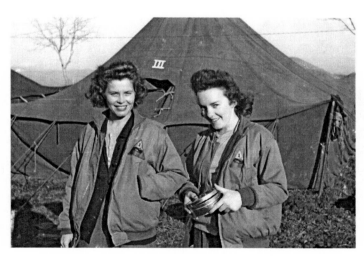

Nurses Ziegler and Haase of the Eleventh Field

cerned. We haven't had a patient our last two shifts. However, we've had word that there's a push of some kind starting in the morning. Had a little party here this evening—2nd Aux and 11th Field people—wasn't bad. Fitzpatrick here. He's going home on compassionate leave—wife is sick. Miss Ziegler of 11th Field is going home tomorrow on month's leave—but there's still no hope for me.

Sunday, October 15, 1944

9:15 Sunday night and work is piling up fast. Have three tables going so we may be called at midnight. To bed now just in case. The 442nd Infantry Regiment (American-born Japs) are coming in Bruyeres from the north and we're getting their casualties. One just died in the shock tent and another on the table. Sort of a mixed-up business—they're dying for a country that is fighting like hell to put their people's land out of existence.

Monday, October 16, 1944

Work has been heavy last night and today but seems to be letting up now. Yesterday as one attack started off they came face-to-face with a Jerry attack. Jerry is always doing that—we attack and he has one for the same time. Mail today—first in a while—got six letters from Marion, all of which were good. First I've had from her saying that she had heard from me in France—a long time to wait. She mentioned Dave Reidy wounded in France. It seems that there is a constant trickle of names dead, missing in action, or wounded—names of fellows I know.

Tuesday, October 17, 1944

Worked until 5:30 this a.m. on one guy and then he died at 11:00 (but he really had no right to live the way he was frapped up) [case 200].

> Case 200. General condition on admission extremely poor. B.P. 0/0. No palpable pulse at wrist. Breathing shallow and automatic. Colon herniating through abdominal wound. This portion of colon was transected. Lung fields moist.

Slept 'til noon but I didn't get much sleep at that—too much noise here. Weather still wet but not too bad. Most all the cases we're getting now are from the 442nd Infantry—Jap-American soldiers. They're a tough-looking crew and are good patients.

Wednesday, October 18, 1944

Supposedly another push on Bruyeres was started this morning. We did two cases this evening and more are coming in. Getting some Jerry prisoners. A case I did had a penetrating wound of the epigastrium—the missile going on thru and partly out his left flank, denting a grenade which we removed from his left pocket. Almost, I'd say. I'm keeping the slug— also I'll paste in a couple of stamps he had on him.

Thursday, October 19, 1944

Did a case this afternoon but work is slow generally. Kaplan returned from our headquarters at Epinal and brought some mail for me—four from Marion which were good—mail, a wonderful buildup but oh, how lonely and anxious I feel after reading it.

Had a series of air raids in this vicinity tonight but nothing much. Still lots of artillery flying around.

Bruyeres fell today—seven miles from here so we'll be moving soon.

Friday, October 20, 1944

Got busy here at noon and had quite a rush for a while. We did three bellies while Brewer's team was doing one. Chunn lost a thoracotomy (bleeding internal mesenteric artery). A couple of Jerries that were 20 hours old and had marked peritonitis.

Sun out for a change—beautiful fall day, but it's wasted. The rain is more in line with my feelings—will be until I get home.

Saturday, October 21, 1944

Busy all afternoon and evening. Had a guy who had no right to live with all he had, but he survived operation [case 206].

> Case 206. T. K. NMI Pfc. 39084564 Age 25 442 inf.
>
> | Injured | 1100 hrs. | 21 Oct 44 | Shell frag. |
> |---|---|---|---|
> | 3rd Bn Aid Sta | 1100 hrs. | Sulf dressing | 2 units plasma |
> | 886 Coll Co | 1225 hrs. | Rx none | |
> | Clr. Sta 111th Med Bn | 1300 hrs. | 1 cc T.T. | |
> | 11th Field Hosp. | 1300 hrs. | | |
>
> Gen'l condition on admission extremely poor. B.P. 0/0. Pulse imperceptible.
> Abdomen rigid and tender
> Diagnosis: S.F.W., perf., abdominal sv

Preop Rx.:
1320 hrs. B.P. 0/0 plasma started.
1330 M.S. gr $^1/_6$ atropine gr $^1/_{100}$ IV 25,000 units of Penicillin.
1335 hrs. 2nd unit of plasma. 1350 hrs. 500 cc blood.
1445 hrs. B.P. 100/50 500 cc blood.
1530 hrs. B.P. 104/66 P. 130 500 cc blood.
1545 hrs. B.P. 70/40 P. 120.

Wd. of left costophrenic area with eviscerated omentum. Patient was never out of shock and after 1500 cc of blood B.P. still 70/30 P 120 it was thought advisable to start surgery. Pt. on side. Wd. of rt. lower lateral thorax debrided and incision extended down over abdomen. Left thoracic cavity had not been opened. Abdomen full of blood. Spleen was shattered. Splenectomy done and bleeding controlled. Splenic flexure of colon in shreds. Mobilized and delivered thru stab wd. of left upper rectus. Bowel resected over clamps. Clamps left on bowel ends as double barrel colostomy. Jejunum was site of four complete transections—three feet resected. End to end anastomoses.

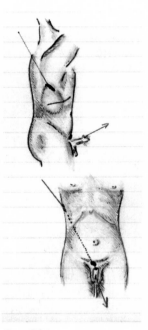

Case 206

Missile passed out of peritoneal cavity thru left lower rectus. Passed over bladder dome and out of abdominal wall at base of Penis. Then into penis and along shaft passing out at the glans penis. Catheter had been passed into bladder from below and sutured in place. Supra pubic cystostomy done. Shaft and glans penis reconstructed. Three retention sutures through all layers of incision. Abdomen closed in layers. 4000 cc blood pre and during operation. Fractured 10th rib and cartilage resected. B.P. 70/30 P. 120 at end of operation.

26-Oct 44 Progress has been excellent. Was never anything but mentally sharp. Colostomy working. Urine clear. Doing very well. T 100 P 90 R 24

28-Oct-44 Eating reg. diet. Suprapubic catheter out. Colostomy working well.

Party at the quarters but like the last one we're on call. They had delicious steak sandwiches, however, of which I had two.

Somebody has an in with a French meat house. First decent steak I've had in months. Some talk over at the clearing station of moving to Bruyeres very soon. Hate to move out of this comfortable place and back into tents.

Sunday, October 22, 1944

Slept thru 'til 11 a.m.—got up just in time to make Mass. Frapped-up case we did last night is still alive tonight and not doing too badly. Hitched down to Remiremont to the 10th Field today but all our teams had left except Ken Lowry—they're holding there. French have moved in there, replacing the 3rd Division.

Weather is looking toward winter—it actually looked like snow today.

Monday, October 23, 1944

Clearing station moving tomorrow so we'll probably be moving out of here this week—to Bruyeres.

On all day but didn't get a case 'til after supper, but that one case took us until 11:00. He was completely wounded if any soldier ever was [case 207].

Case 207. Diagnosis: Shell fragment wds. multiple pen. and perf. abd., rt; arm, rt.; shoulder, rt and left; buttocks; Lumbodorsal region; rt and left thighs; rt and left legs; left ankle sv.

Raining, as per usual—getting cold, too, and real winter isn't far off. I hate to think of being here until next spring or summer but I'm sure that that's my lot. At this point I feel like quitting but that's not possible—nothing to do but just keep going and hoping and wishing.

Wednesday, October 25, 1944

Bruyeres is still under rather heavy artillery fire so we can't move until it quiets down. Had two cases this afternoon. The last one I did and it was a dilly—sacral penetration with fragment coming out at the umbilicus [case 209].

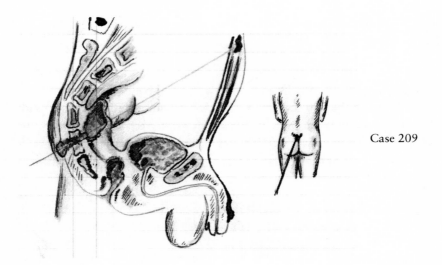

Case 209

Work isn't heavy now, but it's steady. First case we did was a medic from the 111th Medical Battalion alongside of us here. One company of 141 was cut off two days ago and hasn't been heard of since.

Radio tonight told of great naval battles in the Philippine seas. The war is greener everywhere but here. And here it's just tough going every day.

October 26, 1944

This starts my third book since I first began writing one rainy day at Kilmer.

It's already the 27th, 3 a.m.—just finished—a thoracotomy and laparotomy on a fellow. Had two cases after supper which have kept us busy 'til now. We've had great luck with our cases recently and even those we were certain were fatally wounded have lived. Some of the other teams are having a bad series.

Saturday, October 28, 1944

Sullivan here this a.m. I may be moved into a spot where I'd have a team of my own but not definite yet. Don't know whether I should take it or not—it's a big responsibility and I'll have a thousand worries over which I'll stew constantly. One thing it will do is give me responsibility and that's what I need now. Being with G. has been an education but at times a little trying. I profited no end by our association.

Sunday, October 29, 1944

Just finished our second case and it's after midnight. I'm in for a full dusk to dawn of work 'cause shock is still full. Just had a grilled cheese sandwich (Madding and Curtiss live in the diet kitchen of this place and have electric appliances). Somehow or other the cases we're getting are more severely wounded than previously. These two tonight were really surgical gymnastics 'cause they can't possibly survive. Weather turning cold but nice for change. Heavy frost this morning. Rumor here this evening says that the 3rd Division has broken through the German line and is going full blast toward Strasbourg.

Monday, October 30, 1944

Worked 'til after breakfast this morning then slept 'til 2. Colonel Berry (7th Army surgical consultant) [Frank B. Berry, formerly chief of Surgical Service, Ninth Evacuation Hospital] here. All our cases of last night going OK. One [case 215] is amazing but is doomed, I'm afraid.

> Case 215. Diagnosis: Perf G.S.W., Lumbar dorsal region, right exit thru abd. cavity. (Kidney, Liver, duodenum, colon.) F.C.C. radius right. Perf. wd. right forearm. Patient died on 8th post-operative day.

No word yet as to my prospective change. I'm in a stew.

Tuesday, October 31, 1944

Work is fairly heavy now. Started at 4 this afternoon and here it looks like an all-night session. No mail in days from Marion. Two V-mails from Mom today. At this point I think I should record that I feel as low as a snake. There's no sign of my getting home until the middle of next year. That's so awfully far away. At least we're having beautiful weather now.

Wednesday, November 1, 1944

Truck called for me early this morning as I was busy on the ward to take me here—to Grandvillier to 10th Field Hospital. I'm now chief of G.S. No. 26,[7] Ken Lowry's team—he's gone to 23rd Station Hospital. I have a terrible feeling in my stomach—this responsibility is going to be my undoing. I did big cases with Gordon but it was something to have him across the table from me. Now I must make the decisions. There are many things I could write about the past year or more with G., but suffice it to say it has been a real education for me. I hope and pray I do a good job now.

Thursday, November 2, 1944

We went on call at 4 p.m. yesterday and had two cases last night. Got in bed at 3:30. One chest case was a problem and I'm not sure that I did right by the boy. He's got a temperature of 102 tonight and now I'm in a stew. [He later noted in his medical journal: "Both patients evacuated on 11/11/44 in good condition."] I hope I don't have to worry constantly about these cases. I feel that when I get a few under my belt I'll be all right. Today I start the first day of my third year overseas—I feel like the devil, too. I'd do just about anything to get home. But what to do?

Friday, November 3, 1944

It's really Saturday morning—we started work after supper. Did two cases that were really pips. And when I was into each one I was wishing that I was miles away. I don't know if I can keep up with this job—it worries hell out of me constantly. A great experience but it's no fun. Weather is lousy—and again I've got water under my cot. This tent business is no fun.

Saturday, November 4, 1944

My thoracotomy died this morning and at post I found no reason for his death. As somebody said, these shells were meant to kill and sometimes they do. Mail came up from headquarters today and I got six from Marion, which helped very much. A couple from Ethel telling me all about my wonderful wife and kids—and how she can tell it. Rumors around today that this group of 2nd Aux in France is to be detached from headquarters in Italy. Might mean a good break for me.

Sunday, November 5, 1944

Got thru the night without a call and almost all day. Did a bilateral fractured femur just before dinner—which wasn't much of a job. Weather nice again—beautiful moon out tonight which in the soft darkness makes me almost feel that home and Marion aren't too far away. The awful loneliness of this place is somehow crowded out by the soft glow of moonlight that, as it shines here, will shine there tomorrow.

Monday, November 6, 1944

New schedule—on 12, off 24. We were on all day and finally got a case at 5:00. Fellow had a belly full of jejunal contents and took us a couple hours to do. Getting cold and blowing. Every minute I think the tent is about to take off and leave us. Sully up today. New division coming in the line here—the 100th, and one platoon of this field hospital is gonna be detached to them. So may be moving again today or tomorrow.

Tuesday, November 7, 1944

Election Day—news is going to broadcast over 7th Army station at 4 a.m. Go on call at 8 tonight but things are very quiet. Still raining and the mud is getting awfully thick. This is really a very monotonous existence—either in the ward or in your tent. The floor of the tent is muddy— my feet are wet and I'm lonesome!

Wednesday, November 8, 1944

Roosevelt for four more years. Now that I voted for him I can't tell why I did. Purely selfish motive. I just think he'll get the war over sooner. Got thru the night without a case. My other cases are doing OK. I'm not as afraid of this job as I was when I first took it.

Thursday, November 9, 1944

Did a tough case this a.m. and I'm having a time keeping him alive. I fear he's been mortally wounded but we'll see. Had liver, stomach, colon, spleen, jejunum, and kidney [case 225].

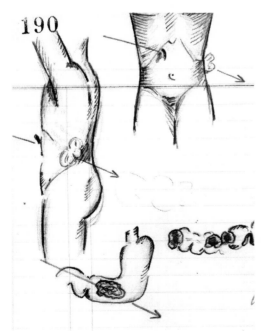

Case 225

Case 225. G.C. Sgt. 31321476 Age 19 B.P. 7th Inf.

Injured 0530 hrs. 9 Nov. 44 Shell frag.

1st Bn Aid Sta 7th Inf   0730 hrs. Sulf crystals dressing M.S. gr ½

Co A Coll   0950 hrs.

Clr. Sta. 3rd Med Bn 0800 hrs.

10th Field Hosp.   0830 hrs.

Gen'l condition on admission poor although B.P. was 100/60. Abd.
    was rigid & tender ++++. Colon herniating thru left flank exit
    wd. Liver herniating thru entrance wd. right upper abdomen.
    Catheterized urine contained blood. Pulse 160.

Diagnosis: S.F.W. perf. thoraco abdominal left, sv. incurred 0530 hrs.
    near Jaques, France.

Preop Rx: Plasma U TT Blood 500 cc (O). Penicillin 25,000 units.
    T.T. ½ cc. Atropine 1/100 I.V. B.P. 0850 hrs. was 110/60.

B.P. dropped to 80/50 while in transit. Shock—Xray—to O.R. Rose
    to 110/60 before induction. During induction dropped to 80/50 to
    50/40 to 0/0.

1000 hrs.	110/60	P. 160	Endotracheal E & O2	blood from shock running Plasma unit I
1015 hrs.	50/40	P. 140		
1030 hrs.	50/40	P. 140	500 cc blood (O)	Pt turned semi rt side
1040 hrs.	0/0			Operation started.
1100 hrs.	0/0		1000 5% glucose in saline	
1130 hrs.	50/40		Plasma U I (new)	Blood 500 cc (O).
1200 hrs.	90/50		Plasma U I	
1230 hrs.	90/50	P. 140		
1245 hrs.	100/50	P. 130		
1300 hrs.	100/50			
1330 hrs.	110/60		Blood 500 cc (O)	
1340 hrs.	100/60	P. 128		op ended.

Pt. turned on right side so as to make left abd. and flank accessi-
ble. Entire abdomen prepared. Colon herniating thru wd. of exit.
Liver herniating thru wd. of entrance. Abdomen opened thru left
upper left rectus incision. Abd. full of blood, fecal material, and

stomach contents. Leading edge left and right lobe liver site of fracture laceration. Anterior and posterior surface of stomach perforated—several inches in diameter—Jejunum transected 7 inches from Lig. of Treitz. Left half transverse colon, splenic flexure and proximal portion of descending colon transected several times and perforated. Spleen has minimal laceration at lower pole. Kidney not lacerated but contused.

Herniating colon returned to peritoneal cavity. Left half transverse colon, splenic flexure and part of proximal descending resected. Spica colostomy formed. Jejunum anastomosed—end to end. Large perforations of stomach closed transversely. Large fragments of liver which were almost completely detached were excised and removed. Liver fracture site drained. Morison's pouch drained—1 penrose drain & 1 penrose cigarette drain. Costophrenic sinus left had been opened by missile and sucked as this area was exposed. Closed with two silk mattress sutures tied on outside over a gauze roll. Sucking controlled. Large peritoneal defect in left flank at 10th rib closed from within—this area from which colon was resected was drained. 10 gms. sulf into peritoneal cavity. Four retention sutures through all layers. Abdomen closed in layers. Penrose drain down to posterior rectus fascia. Wd. of entrance debrided. Muscle defect closed. Wd. of exit debrided. Muscle dark brown and infiltrated with fecal material. Distal lower portion of 10th rib excised. Muscle defect closed. Chest aspirated. Blood & air recovered. Intercostal chest tube inserted in 9th interspace connected to water trap.

9 Nov 2000 hrs. Reacted at 5 p.m. B.P. full at 6 p.m. P. rapid. 4:30 p.m. 500 cc O blood. Developed urticaria at 5:15. Ephedrine SO4 gr $^3/_8$ ordered by Capt Wm Edwards in my absence. 500 cc blood A at 6:00 p.m. Plasma 2 units. 500 cc glucose in saline following blood. Caffeine with sodium benzoate.

Lots of mail today, which makes me happy but sad afterward—got a picture of Paulie and Joanie and Ruthie and I could hardly believe my eyes, they've grown so. Looked wonderful to me. First snow of the year fell today—melted as fast as it fell.

Friday, November 10, 1944
My man is about to quit—second death I've had here. Good-looking kid,

six foot, age 19. He's irrational but he's got one good idea—he keeps repeating—Get me home, please!

10 Nov

M.S. gr $^{1}/_{6}$ 2 a.m.

Blood 500 cc A 3 a.m. followed by 500 cc 5% glucose in saline. B.P. at 3 a.m. 82/64.

8 a.m. B.P. 96/78. Plasma 2 units.

10 a.m. B.P. 110/70.

10:30 a.m. B.P. 96/70 P. 144.

11:15 a.m. 500 cc blood A followed by 300 cc glucose in saline.

Noon B.P. 100/78 P. 144.

1 p.m. 1000 cc glucose in water.

1:30 p.m. B.P. 110/70.

2 p.m. water trap changed. Drained 300 cc.

2:30 p.m. B.P. 100/60 P 152.

3:30 p.m. B.P. 110/80 P. 152 R. 40

4:30 B.P. 110/70. Catheterized—50 cc urine (Total since op 200cc bloody urine).

5:15 p.m. out of shock position.

5:30 p.m. B.P. 100/60.

6:30 84/60 5% glucose in water 1000 cc subcutaneous.

7:30 p.m. Started on sodium citrate 2.5% I.V. q 6 hrs. 300cc 1st dose.
    7:30 p.m. B.P. 80/60 P. 150. Chest dry.

3rd Medics pulled out this morning and were replaced by the clearing station of the 103rd Division, fresh from the States. They're an ambitious, cocky bunch but they'll learn. We're on call tonight—hope it's quiet.

Saturday, November 11, 1944

Thought maybe the war would end today—the last one did—but no such luck.

My boy C. died today. We worked hard on him but to no avail. Some family is gonna get a blow in a few weeks' time, but such is war.

11 Nov. 44. Gen'l condition very poor. Still not moist though I was called by nurse at 4 a.m. because "he sounded wet." B.P. 80/60 P. 152. Sodium citrate continued. Catheterized. 25 cc dark brown fluid. Acid reaction. Ht. 53. Hb 18/100. Plasma P. 1023. Blood sp. gr. ok. 1062.

1600 hrs. Expired.—had isolated convulsive movements just prior to death. Postem mortem revealed a moderate amount of generalized peritonitis. All suture lines intact. 200 cc fluid in each pleural cavity. Kidneys grossly neg. kidney, liver, spleen, lung, tissue sent to 1st Med. Lab.

Sully up here today—we're being augmented by teams from another surgical group so work will be a little lighter. They're just arriving from the States. Such flaunting of experience that will be done.

3rd Army seems to be making great gains between Metz and Nancy. Story is that this is the breakthrough.

Monday, November 13, 1944

Had my third death—thought it was a pulmonary embolus but was wrong—fellow had a foul pelvic infection.

Drove over to Bruyeres to the 11th Field; they're set up in buildings, steam heat, and all—very comfortable. It was snowing hard when we woke up this morning and everything was covered—very pretty but not to look at from a tent. I get my feet wet several times a day—fortunately I have two pair of shoes—I wear one and keep a pair by the fire.

Thursday, November 16, 1944

I'm writing this 10 a.m. of Friday, November 17. We were on call all night and worked until just now. Did only two cases, but they were tough and I had one hell of a time, particularly with the last one. I had to mobilize his splenic flexure and I just couldn't get it out. Finally I got my colostomy made but it was tight as all get out and I'm not sure if it's gonna take.

Got a lot of mail yesterday—nine from Marion—good getting it but oh, how much more lonesome I get afterward. I'm sick of war, mud, and cold; sick of being away from my family; sick of seeing healthy strong bodies shot so full of holes. I'm ready to call it quits right now—to bed.

Friday, November 17, 1944

Got a few hours' sleep but I couldn't help worrying about the one case I did during the previous night. Work coming in all day. 103rd Division is fighting around St. Die. According to the radio, there are pushes on all up and down the line. The 9th and 1st Armies are fighting in Germany east of Aachen and are making good progress. Weather was warm—sky clear—the air force was out in great strength going over here all day. Got our whiskey ration today and five of us drank my bottle—it chases the worries and blues away—just a little glow. How wonderful it would be now to have Marion with me—here or anyplace in the world. It would make no difference where 'cause for the time that place would be heaven.

Saturday, November 18, 1944

Moved today to Baccarat with Major Kennedy's platoon of 10th Field. We're supporting the 2nd French Armored Division. Just two teams here—Frosty Lowry and our team, so if there's any work at all, we'll be pretty rushed. This town was pretty well shot up. There's a church that has nothing left standing but a few pieces of wall. They say this armored division just came in here with all guns blazing and just shot hell out of the place. This building we're in was a German hospital. Place is all marked with Jerry signs.

Sunday, November 19, 1944

My birthday—again—they seem to be flying by. This was my third one overseas and I hope and pray my last one—but I'm not too sure it will be. Started a case right after breakfast and worked through 'til 8:30 this evening—didn't even get to Mass. Had some good cases. Colonel Berry by here this afternoon and when he saw how busy we were he sent a third team up—Don Williams [Donald B. Williams, thoracic surgeon].[8]

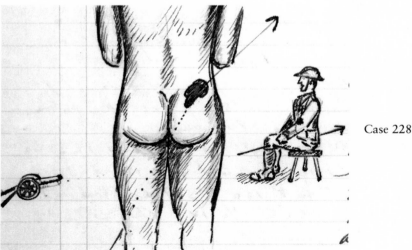

Case 228

Monday, November 20, 1944

Like everything else that's any good, this very pleasant stay has come to an abrupt end. Lowry's team are leaving tomorrow with the 57th Field for Saarburg, still behind the 2nd French Armored. Major Kennedy has an excellent setup here—was just too good to last. Saarburg is way out on a salient and is just a little far out for me. French broke thru to Rhine below Belfort.

Tuesday, November 21, 1944

Started for Saarburg early this morning after working 'til 2 a.m. Got as far as Blamont—halfway—and waited there for several hours, only to have to turn back. A bridge was out and the town was still in question. Blamont had been shelled Sunday afternoon and it was almost completely demolished—by American artillery. In one yard in an air raid shelter there were six coffins, several with the lids open showing a couple mangled bodies. A Jerry was lying over in one ditch—awfully dead. The people on the street didn't speak or smile—they just looked straight ahead as they passed. Can sort of see their point of view. Staying tonight with Major Kennedy's platoon of 10th Field.

Wednesday, November 22, 1944

Left at 9 this morning and arrived here in Saarburg at noon—only 30 kilometers but the traffic was very heavy—We're set up in an old school building. Last night it was the C.P. for a battalion of the 44th Division—the night before Jerries lived in it. Tonight it's a hospital. Three shells struck the building last night—hope that was the last. This field hospital is spanking new and they don't know anything about this work, all of which makes its worse for us.

Thursday, November 23, 1944, Thanksgiving

Had a very unpleasant night. Saarburg was shelled and I'll swear they sounded as if they were coming in the room with us. All the 57th personnel headed down cellar but like nuts we stayed in bed.

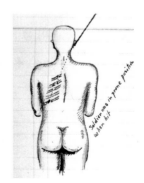

Did one case today, a Jerry, a bullet went in his right ear and ended up in his left chest—not half as bad as it sounds [case 232].

Had an excellent turkey dinner, much to my surprise. Our French armored division is now in

Case 232

Strasbourg, so tomorrow or the next day we're going in there. They'll get us captured yet.

Friday, November 24, 1944

Moving again to Strasbourg in the morning. The French have the bridge over the Rhine and this evening were seven miles into Germany and going ahead quite fast.

Colonel Forsee and Major Sullivan here today making their rounds—no news. Walked around town a little this morning and I'm amazed at how different the people here appear—they're pure German, I'm sure, and certainly have little time for us.

Saturday, November 25, 1944

Strasbourg—after much dickering we finally left Saarburg after lunch and headed north. Sunshine, rain, and rainbows chased us all the way. Saw many Jerry strong points that had been knocked out, minefields, trenches, etc. Came through the Saverne Gap, which tonight B.B.C. says is under counterattack. The towns we passed through are neater and cleaner than anything we've previously seen. The answer is simple—they're German. Strasbourg is a town of 97,000—on the Rhine, and from the brief glimpse I've had of it, it seems to be a very modern town. We're set up in one building of the Grand Hospital Civil and we're set up like kings. Best that we've ever had. There are many German doctors here and they've been fairly friendly. Brott talks German so tonight one of the younger M.D.s took us through several blocks. Met the professor of surgery Dr. Zukschwerdt and through Brott talked with him for an hour. The wing we were in was staffed by German officers and nurses and they were operating on Jerries. This afternoon saw several Jerry doctors walking around here in well-kept and classy uniforms. I'm wondering right now just who is whose prisoner. Strasbourg is ours but the bridges over the river are still in German hands. There are hundreds of tanks spread throughout the city, strategically placed, and patrols wander about. It's a peculiar situation. We're in a Kraut nest all right.

Sunday, November 26, 1944

There's lots of gunfire going around here, most of which is small arms but nobody seems to be getting hurt. At least not the French, so slept thru the night without a call. Went to Mass this a.m. in a church on the hospital grounds—it was a high Mass in which not only the choir but all the congregation sang the responses and did it well. Hymns were sung both in French and German. Although this is French territory the people here are Germans.

It's interesting to hear the B.B.C. talk of the fighting in this area. Last night they told of a heavy Jerry counterattack in the Saverne Gap through the Vosges Mountains—we had come through there about four p.m. They told today of the Jerries holding the bridges over the Rhine—and they do. The city now is approximately 90% taken. Some one of these nights they're gonna blow these bridges and it will just about blast me out of bed. Still considerable sniping going on in town. Two French officers were killed near here last night. Needless to say, come dark we stay indoors. There's rumor going about that the Jerries are gonna try and take Strasbourg back again—that would be interesting but it doesn't worry me in the least.

Monday, November 27, 1944

Still no work from the French but supposedly they're attacking south tomorrow along the Rhine to get the 50,000 Jerries that are between here and Mulhouse. The French 1st Army is coming up from the south and American troops will come in from the Vosges Mountains. We're the cork in the bottle 'cause the bridges over which they'll try to cross the Rhine are here at Strasbourg.

Tuesday, November 28, 1944

Still no wounded Frenchmen—the radio from London says the French are pushing south but evidently we're having very few casualties. News is scant and progress is even less, but I don't think it will be long before we go over the Rhine. Fairly noisy around here today but nothing more.

Gordon and Childs [Samuel B. Childs, assistant general surgeon and Kennedy's replacement on GS #6] hitched up here today and were quite impressed with the place—they were also very impressed with the "hotness" of the town and were anxious to get out before dark—which they did.

Did a small case at 0100 hours this morning that's all I've done since I arrived.

Wednesday, November 29, 1944

Tomorrow we go back to Saverne to follow up the 45th Division on another tack. This was a beautiful setup and never will we meet it again. Some talk of the 10th Field moving in here—will kill me to see the other 2nd Aux take over.

Walked into Strasbourg this afternoon just to take a quick look around. It was fairly well frapped up. No people on the streets; all stores closed—just a few M.P.s around—everything looks and reads very German. Occasional shots—a few 90s, but everything else is very quiet. The Germans still hold the bridges but we didn't walk down there to see.

Did a case at 4 this morning—through and through the flank. Doing OK.

Thursday, November 30, 1944

Was called last night at 1 and we worked 'til breakfast. Didn't get any sleep today. The hospital moved out this morning, leaving several sick patients to be taken care of by corpsmen with little or no supplies. A Jerry I did—and who is gonna die—was wounded here in Strasbourg. He's been sniping in the town for the past five days and was finally caught. Slug went in his belly and out his back. I guess it's a deserved fate—at least no one here has any sympathy for him.

10th Field moving in here tomorrow to take our place behind the French 2nd Armored Division.

Friday, December 1, 1944

Were all set to go at 8 this a.m. but vehicles didn't appear 'til 3 p.m. 10th Field—Major Beatty's platoon with Fish attached moved in the meantime to our once-nice spot. The drive back thru the Saverne pass was difficult—a heavy fog and black driving, meeting numerous truck convoys, made it so. We almost hit the ditch several times. Finally made Saarburg at 9 p.m. Staging here with 57th headquarters tonight and tomorrow we'll join Rosenberg's platoon behind the 100th Division.

Saturday, December 2, 1944

Up at 7 to get an early start but didn't get away 'til almost noon. Set up west of Saverne near the town of Rauweiller with the 100th Clearing Station. Back in tents in a muddy field—cold, wet, and poorly set up. It's sort of difficult to come out of nice buildings and find yourself in a tent—and we'll be in tents going in the direction we are. Heard a new rumor today—Jerry prisoners are quoted as saying that all firing will stop on December 5 (it's now December 3).

Sunday, December 3, 1944

Blowing and raining outside to beat all hell—has been all day and this area is fast turning into a mud puddle. To top things off, the generator gave up the ghost so we're seeing by a candlepower.

This field hospital deserves some credit for trying, but that's all—it takes them days to set up and then they usually get it backwards on the first try.

Mass this morning over in the clearing station (100th Division). Even they are new. I guess it's about time the 2nd Aux was sent home 'cause the old and new don't mix over here.

Few cases coming in but we're not catching them on our shift.

Monday, December 4, 1944

Getting to bed about 1 p.m. Did a chest case this morning and a thoraco-abdominal this afternoon and evening. Work is steady now but things are difficult here because of the inefficiency of this field hospital. Lights go out right in the middle of things—things are usually done backwards, etc. Sully here this morning and we cried on his shoulder but he doesn't give much sympathy. I guess too many people are crying on his shoulder. This Major Barrett of the 1st Aux is quite a person—he's a regular little Napoleon but without a command. Obviously hasn't seen any of this work before but he still tries to talk as if he has.

Tuesday, December 5, 1944

Fairly busy today—did two cases—a belly and a chest. Major Barrett, our friend, had one die on the table. The poor guy tries to put up such a front and won't admit that he hasn't seen anything like this previously.

Lots of air activity here today. Several Me 109s were strafing along this road. Tanks going up all day by the thousands. Weather still foul—raining and lots of mud. Radio tells of another crossing of the river Saar.

Wednesday, December 6, 1944

New plan for us—at least a move is certain in a day or two—going behind some armored division. There's no chance of ever getting tired of one spot in this organization. Work coming in slowly but steadily. Doing two cases a day and that's plenty—have a chest now that is worrying me enough for a dozen cases. War news slow—everybody "patrolling" but the 3rd Army—they seem to be continuously on the move—are across the Saar in several places now in strength. Never saw so much armored stuff—lined up the road for miles—all marked by a bright orange red flag draped across their top for aircraft identification. No air activity around here, however.

Thursday, December 7, 1944

Orders to move tomorrow. Barrett staying as a holding company—(my poor patients). Two new surgical teams, 1st Aux, to join us at Carney's platoon. If Carney is in the field, we'll have a terrific time 'cause in buildings he was lousy. Did a thoraco-abdominal tonight—rather simple but interesting. Another one of those bleeding belly walls into peritoneal cavity.

Raining all day and the mud is getting deeper.

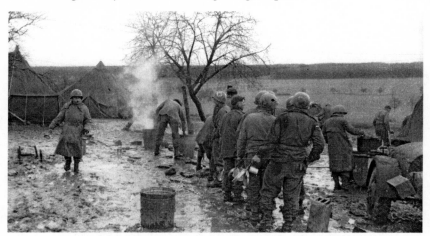

Chow line in the mud near Rauwiller, France. "The Group was fortunate in having well trained cooks but the repeated issue of Vienna sausage, spam, chili-con-carne, dehydrated potatoes, beets, carrots and powdered eggs severely taxed their ingenuity in the preparation of appetizing foods" (*Forward Surgery of the Severely Wounded: A History of the Activities of the 2nd Auxiliary Surgical Group*, 831).

Friday, December 8, 1944

Sat around 'til 3 in the afternoon waiting for the trucks to pick us up. Finally got away after supper and got as far as Saverne. Found out at the 57th Field Hospital headquarters that the road had been shelled out and was difficult to drive over in the black so we're staying here for the night. This is another *Krankenhaus* [hospital] and was quite a nice place. Headquarters outfits always have a habit of finding a nice place to set up. Leave for Bauxweiller in the a.m.

Saturday, December 9, 1944

Arrived here at 10 this a.m. The road would have been a son of a gun to get by in the dark. This town is a quaint little place and hardly touched by the war. The houses are all roof and numerous beams and are very picturesque. Everything is neat and clean.

The hospital unit is set up in what had been a Jerry headquarters—they didn't leave it in any too good a condition—dirty—but our troops do the same thing. Cantlon's team came here last night—that gives us three 2nd Aux.

Walked into the town after lunch just looking around. Nothing open since it was Saturday afternoon, but we did get into a hotel thru the back door—a very clean, quaint-looking place which had already been taken over by some outfit. Had a couple beers which weren't too bad but still not too much like beer. They have no hops in Germany.

I mentioned a Dr. Busee—we met him at Strasbourg—earlier in these pages. I learned from Cantlon today that he was picked up and held—turned out to be a Nazi.

Sunday, December 10, 1944

Big, dumb, simple Major Tom Carney called me at 4:30 a.m. to see a case but it was nothing. Mass at 9 a.m. in the clearing station and to Communion. Mass was read downtown in a hall on the village square. We sang our heads off—not good but loud. I wonder what these people thought of soldiers that go to church and pray. Did one case this afternoon. We go on again at midnight and I suspect we'll be busy—VI Corps started a push today along its entire front and that means business for us. Frosty had a chest case die on the table after he had worked on him for four hours—very discouraging, to say the least.

Monday, December 11, 1944

The rush of casualties we were supposed to get never came—just a few. The 45th Division took its objective without much trouble. They're now four miles from the Siegfried line. The clearing station is moving up and another platoon of this hospital is going with them so we'll go too.

Saw two of our bombers and a fighter crash today just behind the hill over to our left. They made weird noises and then plunged to the ground. Explosions and three large columns of smoke jumped out of the earth as they hit.

Tuesday, December 12, 1944

Didn't get much sleep last night. Had a case come in at 12 for which I was prematurely called. It was hours before I had X-rays, etc. then decided to evacuate him—got to bed at 3. Packed up this morning and right after lunch we started out. As usual things were tarfu and we had no ambulance for personnel. I fortunately got a ride in Father Carney's jeep. This town, Oberbronn, is about 12 miles from Bauxweiller but the roads we took were roundabout and poor. Passed several batteries of 155 howitzers and I got a little anxious as far as the chaplain's map reading was concerned. This town is another typical German village, neat and picturesque, built on the side of the hill with a good command of the valley thru which this little part of the war is moving. Haven't had a chance to look around but will tomorrow. They shelled here yesterday but the line has supposedly moved a few miles. However, our phosphorous shells could be seen bursting a few miles ahead of us as we rode into town. The building we're in was a Catholic hospital run by sisters—a very nice place and certainly a pleasant place in which to work.

Only two teams here so if work comes in we'll really be busy.

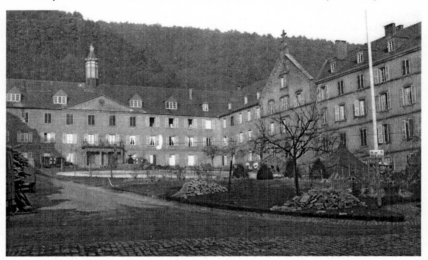

Catholic hospital at Oberbronn, France

Wednesday, December 13, 1944

Work starting to come in. I thought this was going to be a sterile stand but I guess I was wrong. We did two amputations this afternoon—there were three in the shock ward at once—all had their right foot blown off. They were together walking up a railroad track and hit a mine-field. The Jerries are pulling out of these little towns without offer-

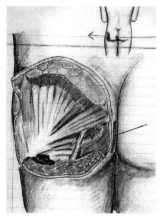

ing any resistance—just leaving minefields and booby traps. Have one more case to do tonight. Fellow had his entire left buttock blown off [case 246; noted later in the medical journal: "Evacuated 12/21/44"].

Thursday, December 14, 1944

Didn't get to bed 'til 3 this morning—got through 'til morning without a call, fortunately. Mary Campbell here this a.m. and took Miss Prather and Miss Lang [Helen L. Lang, nurse][9] away for a couple days—they're going on a leave to Paris. She brought a little mail and I got six from you, Marion. Mail is great but it gives me the "I wanna go homes."

Case 246

Did two cases this evening—both good bellies. I have a lot more confidence in myself now for some reason or other. Most all my cases are doing fairly well, which helps. Father Carney of the 45th Division was in tonight and said the 79th Division is in Germany—that the 45th wasn't pushing now—Maybe we'll get a little rest now.

Friday, December 15, 1944

Writing this 8 a.m. of the 16th. Started working about 24 hours ago and just finished. There's still plenty more work in the shock ward but I can't see straight at this point. We've had some rough cases—one thoracoabdominal of the right side in which the entire liver was herniated into the right chest. Had a transection of the spinal cord too—awful part of his case was that he wasn't a battle casualty—a drunken soldier in the next town shot him.

A little mail today, including Dad's Xmas card—it's a wonderful picture—I've just about looked a hole thru it. Paulie and Joanie and Ruthie are nothing short of perfect and my heart aches to see them. It will be a long while before I do, but as long as I do get home I'll be satisfied. Story around here has the 7th Army in Germany. The 45th Division at the moment is up against the Siegfried line and supposedly it's just like bucking concrete.

Saturday, December 16, 1944

Called at 4:30 p.m. to do a case. But Major "Domo" Barrett's case died on the table and so he did it instead. I did a Jerry tonight—pretty good chest case. Had a transection of the cord die this morning—just as well but not for my records. We're on call tonight but things are quiet so maybe we'll get by.

Sunday, December 17, 1944

Got called at 4 a.m. and didn't finish 'til 9 a.m. Just in time to make Mass in the "Grand" Chapel. It was a high Mass and the sisters sang the response—very nice. I hope we're here Christmas 'cause it will be a beautiful Mass, I'm sure. As things look now we will be. The 45th is practically all in Germany now and is going along OK, but they still aren't up to the Siegfried line.

Weather, strangely enough, is quite pleasant now—not much rain and not very cold.

Monday, December 18, 1944

News from the 1st Army front is very discouraging. Jerry is rearing his ugly head in fine style. Radio silence on the situation at B.B.C. Maybe he'll die after this one last effort—but probably not. Had two cases—last one kept us up 'til 3 a.m. so this is really the 19th. Heard tonight we're gonna move Saturday. That takes us out of here for Christmas—too bad.

["1st Army front" refers to the Battle of the Bulge, the German counteroffensive in Belgium (known as Autumn Mist). In Hitler's fantasy, he hoped to drive through the Ardennes to take Antwerp, thus attaining the dual objectives of denying the Allies a major port from which to supply the advance on Germany and providing a more advanced launching site for the V-2 rocket attacks on Britain. Antwerp having been secured and the Allied forces consequently split in two, he then envisioned wheeling to the north and east to encircle and destroy the British Second and the Canadian First armies.

This offensive met with considerable early success, partly due to surprise and partly due to weather. First, the Allies had considered the Ardennes such an unlikely place for a German attack that the American Fourth and Twenty-Eighth divisions had been rotated there to rest after suffering significant casualties in the battle of the Hurtgen Forest. The third infantry division in the Ardennes—the 106th—had not yet been in combat. The Ninth Armored Division, supporting the 106th, was also inexperienced. Thus the ninety-mile front in the center of the First Army was lightly held by troops that were either unblooded or bloodied.

Second, from the beginning of the offensive on December 16 until the weather cleared on December 26, Allied air superiority had been neutralized. Dominant in the skies over western Europe, the Allies were denied both aerial reconnaissance and the ability to attack the German spearhead.

One of the crucial German intermediate objectives was the key crossroads city of Bastogne. By Christmas, the town, defended by the US Eighty-Second Airborne Division, was completely surrounded. It was here that General Anthony McAuliffe delivered his famous reply to a German demand of surrender: "Nuts."

After the 26th, with clearer weather and air support, successful counterattacks against the German northern flank by Montgomery and against the southern flank by Patton threatened to cut off the German forces, forcing them to withdraw. By January 13, when the British First Airborne made contact with the American Eighty-Second, the Ardennes offensive had been first blunted and then reversed. By January 16, the original front had been restored.]

Tuesday, December 19, 1944

Miss Lang came back from Paris today and from her story it's quite a place to see. Lots of stores, nightclubs, etc. She brought me some perfume which supposedly is the real McCoy—kinda skeptical, however. Cost $30 but $30 in Paris is chicken feed.

There's a move in the air again—supposedly Saturday. We're to hold, however, so maybe we'll be here Xmas. This moving every week gets awfully tiresome after a while—you get in a nice place and just get comfortable when—bang—you've gotta move again. I'll be happy when I get settled down someplace with my family where we can enjoy ourselves.

Wednesday, December 20, 1944

Fried fresh eggs—two of them—for breakfast. A great day in our lives. Must admit they did taste pretty good. Did one case this evening—leaves sort of a bad taste in my mouth, too [case 257]. A large perforating wound of the leg which got all the vessels and much tissue but which left the tibia intact. The kid pleaded with me to save it but it had to come off. I hate to face him in the morning—but I must. Little incidents to be told in a diary—or forgotten, perhaps—but what mountains of importance they are to each individual that owns them.

Still little news from the 1st Army front. I'm afraid we're taking a

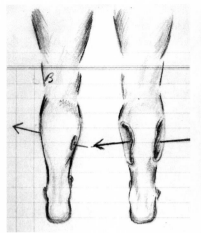
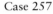

Case 257

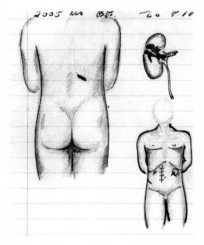

Case 257: post-amputation

licking there—if we hold and stop them, perhaps that will be all that's left of Jerry.

Thursday, December 21, 1944

A one-case day but what a case that was [case 258]. If this fellow gets better I think I'll quit this business and set up for myself. (Nephrectomy, G. bladder, duodenum, liver, and large bowel.)

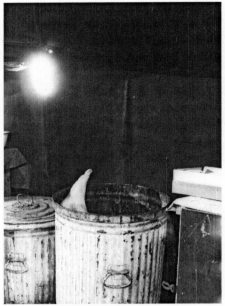

Brott took a couple of patients over to the 117th Evac. Heard over there that a platoon of the 11th Field had been captured in the Colmar section. Lucky I wasn't with them—I have been so much. News from the 1st Army front is still nil, but obviously things are bad. Something else now to prolong this thing.

Case 258

Friday, December 22, 1944

Hurrah, my case of yesterday is fine!

Drove to headquarters this afternoon and picked up some mail. No Xmas mail in at all so I guess it won't get here 'til after the holidays. There's to be a Christmas dinner—we're off that day so we'll go. That story about the 11th Field being captured was just another story, but a Jerry roadblock was built behind them.

Drove down in Rubnitz's [Willard Rubnitz, assistant general surgeon] car today and had to come back in blackout—I'm blind at night. Lots of stuff on the road leading west to 1st Army area—103rd Division, 14th Armored, etc. News from there sounds a little better.

Saturday, December 23, 1944

Moved into new quarters today over in another building and we're really living in fine style. I have a large single bed that is a dream. Two great big duck-down pillows for a comforter. Didn't get in bed 'til about 2 a.m. but once I fell asleep it was heaven (written next morning.)

Did a tough case—fragment entered the back and blew out the duodenum, among other things. Fellow took it all right, however.

Paratroopers were dropped in this vicinity last night. Also, there's another story of the 11th Field Hospital being captured again. News from 1st Army is much improved.

Sunday, December 24, 1944

Just came from midnight Mass. More than ever before I see the real side of Christmas—God's birthday. Stripped of all the things that have made it what it is in the U.S., here in this little mountain German town of Oberbronn [actually in eastern France] it's simply but gloriously God's birthday. The nuns at Mass singing with all their hearts, receiving Communion and returning to their places with black hoods draped over their heads—all seemed to suggest in a clear way how much greater, how much more beautiful that side of Christmas is. Perhaps these lonely Christmases have helped me.

Been busy today—did two pretty big cases finishing the last one just in time to make midnight Mass. This unit had their Christmas party tonight but we didn't have time for it. Going to headquarters for our Christmas tomorrow.

Christmas, 1944

Up for breakfast—got our work done early and then started out in Rubnitz's rattletrap for headquarters. How that thing runs is a mystery—it requires twice as much oil as it does gasoline.

Quite a few teams back so it was a pleasant day—good turkey dinner and good drinks—most everyone had the Christmas "spirits."

Got back here at 7:30 after a blackout drive.

This is my third Christmas overseas—it hardly seems possible but it's true. I pray to God that it's my last 'cause I can't take another.

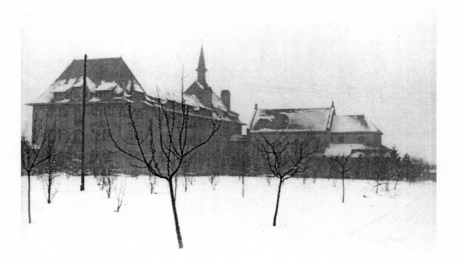

Oberbronn, Christmas, 1944

Tuesday, December 26, 1944

Went to bed at 8:30 last night and didn't get up 'til 10 this morning. Brott got up for breakfast and brought us fried eggs. Breakfast in bed sounds pretty soft. Have a sore throat which has been hanging on for several days. Platoon is moving tomorrow but we're staying on here as a holding company so we'll get another week in our very pleasant quarters. This has been a pretty good stand—had only two deaths out of 19 cases (may have one more cooking) and some of them were real cases.

News from the 1st Army is still not too good but I guess they're getting their breath up there.

Wednesday, December 27, 1944

Just finished a case—it's shortly after midnight and I'm dead tired. We were routed out of bed last night at 1:00 and we worked thru 'til breakfast. Didn't get any sleep today. The hospital platoon tore down early this morning and took off for Lembach, four miles from the German border. They had just finished setting up when they got orders from corps to tear down and come back here. Lucky for us we were the holding company so we just sat tight. This front is awfully uneasy and more uncertain. Lembach was too vulnerable, they say. Even here 155 howitzers are sitting right behind us barking their heads off. As far as I'm concerned it's a question who's winning this war right now.

Thursday, December 28, 1944

Looks like we're gonna be quiet for a while. Nothing in today. Went on a 24-hour off and 24-hour on shift. Drove over to see Gordon and team and had dinner with them. They're fed up with the 57th Field and from the other side of the fence the 57th Field is fed up with them. (There's at least a little bit of good in everybody and if a fellow can "glom" onto that little bit of good and make use of it, he'll very frequently profit by it.) Evacuation hospitals have been pulled back 30 to 40 miles to prevent loss by any sudden breakthrough on Jerry's part—but we sit up here like ducks. Heard over there that Jerry in the Colmar area is massing supplies and men—3rd Division there is being pulled back and dug in on two lines of defense—who's winning now?

Friday, December 29, 1944

Another sterile day—no work except drainage of a subdiaphragmatic abscess. Some artillery outfit has been blasting away all day alongside of us here and each firing shakes the building.

News from the 1st Army front is much improved and we are not on the pushing side. I certainly hope Jerry has spent himself—but I doubt it.

Saturday, December 30, 1944

Finally broke into the mail column today and got six from Marion. Same old story—I look for mail and stew 'til I get some, then when I've read it, I'm more lonesome than ever. The only answer to my problem is to get home, I guess. Walked over to the 240 howitzers that are near us. Got there just in time to see them fire a mission. They were shooting at a German pillbox in the Siegfried line some 14 miles away. They had a telephone connection with an observer who had direct observation on the pillbox. They knocked it out with 20 rounds. Took some pictures of the firing but I'm afraid I missed.

Sunday, December 31, 1944

New Year's Eve—again. I've made some funny statements on the past two New Year's Eves which I won't repeat. Just this—this is my third one overseas and now I'm not a bit confident that it's my last one. (Actually, I believe it is but I won't even let myself hear me say it.)

We worked all night and up 'til noon today. Had an acute fulminating case of gas gangrene—came on in 18 hours. Boy died on the table [case 265]. We had already amputated his left thigh. His right leg was practically nil and he would have lost it. To make matters worse, he had multiple F.B.s in both eyes. Perhaps it's better that he died.

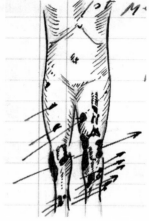

It's snowing here tonight and it's rather pretty—the guns are firing and there's a plane or two buzzing around. Yesterday bombs were dropped near Unit 3 of this hospital— one bomb hit 15 feet from the place. 40 casualties but no hospital personnel.

Case 265

Well, so long, 1944—here's hoping that 1945 sees the end of the war and finds me back with my wonderful, lovely wife and kids.

Monday, January 1, 1945

What you do on New Year's Day, you'll do all year, so the saying goes. Well, tonight we're retreating but I hope we don't do that all year. Jerry is pushing and he's gaining ground. I guess they don't expect to hold this area 'cause we're being moved back. Patients all went out tonight, even two we had just finished operating on—one not yet out of the ether. Nurses left this evening but we're not going 'til early tomorrow morning—but we're all packed and the truck is loaded ready to go. The news from the 1st Army front is good—I guess we're in for a little trouble now. We've never had to retreat, not since Kasserine—it seems funny now— perhaps we won't have to.

Case 267. General condition on admission good (Shock records poor—James was drunk on duty). B.P. supposedly normal. Abd. tender and rigid plus ++. Urine clear. Diagnosis: S.F.W. pen left lumbar region, sv.

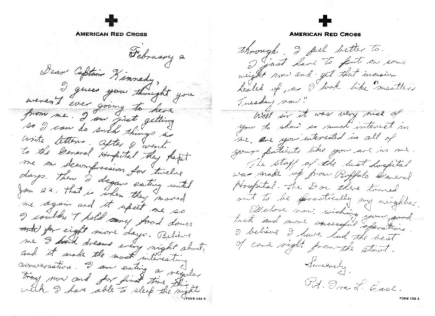

Case 267

Tuesday, January 2, 1945

Moved before dawn out of Oberbronn. Our position was not tenable. Artillery flashing away—tanks set up at crossroads as roadblocks—sort of brought home the fact that we were at home with a war. Moved into buildings just evacuated by the 9th Evacuation Hospital. They pulled back another 50 miles.

Radio is already talking about the German push against the 7th Army. Now Marion and family will be worrying. 2nd Aux headquarters is in the building next door so at least we'll have fresh mail for a while.

It seems that every time we get near the German border we end up in Saarburg—this is the third time we've been set up here.

[As a sort of parallel operation to Autumn Mist, Blaskowitz's Army Group G attacked Patch's Seventh Army in the Saar (Operation North Wind) and enjoyed some brief success, taking a "bulge" on the eastern bank of the Rhine (and forcing the evacuation of Oberbronn). This success was short lived, however, and the Allied line was restored all along the Rhine.]

Wednesday, January 3, 1945

Called at 5 a.m. 10 cases in so we were busy 'til after noon. News on the immediate front is meager. We're pulling back to the Saverne Gap, supposedly to hold there—giving up Strasbourg (and our Oberbronn). (I left my dog tags there so some Jerry will pick them up. Hope they don't record me as a prisoner.)

Thursday, January 4, 1945

Up at 3 a.m. to do a case and worked 'til 5 p.m.—a pretty full day. The cases are 18 to 24 hours old and as a result are in poor shape. Found out at 5 p.m. that we had to move to another building in this group to make room for 132nd Evac. We closed here so we'll have a few free days. The situation in the 7th Army section supposedly improved greatly.

Snowing tonight and it's cold—rather a bad night for the G.I.

Friday, January 5, 1945

Turned my patients over to the 132nd Evac—all in pretty good shape so now we're out of work for a few days. Rode up toward Oberbronn today with Rosenberg and Alcott—started out to get my dog tags that I left there. We got as far as Rothbach, which is some 10 miles beyond Saverne—there we ran into our own mortars that were dug in along the road. We had previously passed tanks that were lined up as artillery. There was an American roadblock set up there and a strong point was being built up. There was supposed to be a patrol of some 30 Jerries coming down the valley some five miles away. Oberbronn, where we had been a few days previously, was once again in "other" hands. Needless to say, we didn't hang around there long.

Got several packages tonight and also the pictures from Uncle Jack and Auntie—they were Kodachrome prints and are wonderful. What a wonderful family I have—and how I'm missing them. (When in hell is this war ever gonna end?)

Sunday, January 7, 1945

Moved up to Pfalsburg today to join B unit of 57th Field. They've been pretty rushed so we're out on loan to them. They're well set up in a school building—heat and lights. Started at 4 on second call and we just finished the last case; it's 12 now so I may get routed out before morning.

Air traffic through the Saverne Gap was stopped yesterday—they say it's under Jerry artillery fire; that's about eight miles from here.

Monday, January 8, 1945

Got called at 3 a.m. so worked until breakfast, then to bed. Back on at midnight so I'm going to bed now. More mail and packages— nice wallet from Marion. News from the western front seems much improved. Only 12 miles between 1st and 3rd Armies, with all but one road supplying Jerry cut. Germans here seem destined to retake Strasbourg. The traffic thru the gap is increased three or four times— all last night tanks went up and today it's been the same way. Cold morning and blowing.

Tuesday, January 9, 1945

Got thru last night without a call. Had one case today—a daisy [case 276]. The largest wound I've yet seen—it practically cut the fellow in

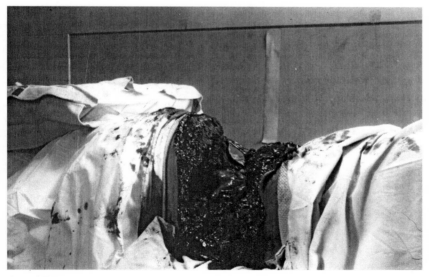

Case 276

two. Pumped blood into him quickly and got his pressure up to 50 systolic—got him on the table but he lasted only a short while.

Still cold and snowing. Went for a walk this afternoon and the countryside covered by snow doesn't look much different from Groton—very white and just now very quiet.

Wednesday, January 10, 1945

Just finished my last case (2 a.m.). Fellow was all frapped up and is without question mortally wounded. First case was eviscerated but he'll do all right [case 277].

Colder and more snow flying today, but the war seems to go on. News from all fronts is much improved.

Thursday, January 11, 1945

Was called at 6 this morning to see that last case—finally died at 4 p.m. He had a foul belly and obviously was mortally wounded. Got a little sleep this afternoon but not much. Its midnight now and we're on first call—there's a case in so I guess we go to work.

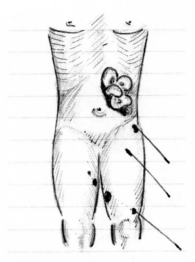

Case 277: "Patient evacuated in good condition, January 16"

Friday, January 12, 1945

Got to bed at 5:30 this morning—did another croaker. The cases I'm getting are of a frapped-up quality. I've lost two already and this fellow is certain to die—discouraging, to say the least. Very cold and more snow.

I wish we could call the war off for the winter so we could all go home. The radio news is improved and although the progress is small, nevertheless, it is progress.

Saturday, January 13, 1945

Had a fairly heavy night but somehow we didn't get called. Cantlon did five cases—he is an eager beaver, I'm afraid. Nothing in all day 'til 4:00 just as we went off call. Got two packages today—one from Ethel and one from Eugene [Kennedy's younger brother]. I'll have to have a trailer to carry all this food around in.

Cold today and our rooms are like ice. Tried to set up a stove but the wind outside is so strong it blows right in the chimney and makes a stove useless.

Sunday, January 14, 1945

Just finished the third case—it's 2 a.m. Every day at about 4 p.m. the cases start coming in. I think the ambulance drivers time it so they'll get here in time for chow.

News from Russia is good for a change—big offensive on the Polish front. Hope it has some real effect.

Wednesday, January 17, 1945

The war news today is all Russian and it's all good. Warsaw fell and on the southern front they're 15 miles from the German border. (How I hope they keep going this time right into Berlin.)

Thursday, January 18, 1945

It's 1:30 and I'm just getting to bed. We did two cases (Brott did a resection, his first, now I'll have to stew till the guy recovers). The second fellow was from a little town near Hershey, Pa.—was like operating on a fellow from home. He's been in the army seven months and landed in Scotland *two weeks* ago. Now he's a casualty—fast work.

Not feeling good—sore throat, etc.

Friday, January 19, 1945

Gordon over this afternoon and stayed for supper. We're gonna write another paper—on liver wounds this time.[10] He has his faults and many people don't like him but he's been a good friend to me and certainly has been a virtual education.

Tuesday, January 23, 1945

A cold, snowy day not much different from yesterday but somehow I feel better tonight for some reason. Several letters from Marion—that's cause enough—a beer ration, a liquor ration, and the Russians are still going strong—170 miles from Berlin. People here are beginning to talk again about the end of the war—but they're not talking very loud. The Jerries took back Haguenau this morning—that's 30 kilometers up this road. Hope they stay up there. Work is practically nil. We haven't done a case in two days or more (which is good—means nobody is getting really hurt).

Sunday, January 28, 1945

Marion's birthday—her third one since I left home—I feel sure that for her next one I'll be home. Still quiet here—no work—but still snowing. Mass and Communion at 1:30 this afternoon. Saw a movie tonight which I saw in the States so long ago that I couldn't recall from one moment to the next just what was coming—*Saboteur*. Planes flying around here all evening.

Friday, February 2, 1945

My spell of no work was broken today—we got a patient today and it was a real case which kept us busy for three hours [case 288]. Fellow was shot by another G.I. as he was coming off outpost duty.

Am being called as a witness tomorrow in a general court-martial in connection with the Chamblin case.

War on 7th Army front still very quiet except in the Colmar area—radio tonight says we are in Colmar.

Quite a number of planes flying around here tonight but nothing dropped.

Saturday, February 3, 1945

Went up to division C.P. today at St. Petit Pierre as a witness in a general court-martial. One of my patients was shot in December by another G.I.—who was drunk—now the fellow is on trial and is charged with murder. I had to testify that Chamblin had died. The defendant has previously been a good soldier—has been wounded three times—he doesn't even remember shooting the fellow—but now he's charged with murder. The sentences that are being handed out now are really rough—one fellow in the 28th Division is being shot for A.W.O.L., and the sentence states that he is to be shot in his own regimental area in the presence of his own regiment—some object lesson, I'd say.

Sunday, February 4, 1945

Up three times during the night—finally did a case at 7 a.m. We're covering the 45th, 103rd ("Nuts" McAuliffe), and the 101st paratroopers. None of them are doing much right now, however. The only real activity in this sector is on the Colmar front.

Tommy Nolan came in to see me this evening—he was the counsel for the defense in the trial yesterday—and told me that his man got off with three years with a recommendation from the court for suspension of sentence. It was a triumph for Nolan.

Monday, February 5, 1945

Heard a sad tale at dinner tonight. There's a nurse in the 11th Field, Skalos is her name, whom I've known since I first joined the 11th in Italy back in 1943. I've seen her off and on as we worked with them at various

March 8

Dear sir;

well here I am at the 43rd General Hospital. I feel pretty good, my hip is pretty sore drains a good bit and is very very odifferous. I got a bottle of blood yesterday that makes 7000 c.c. It seems to me they are changing my oil often these days. I still have my uranary tube. I would sure like to get rid of it but Dr. say not till I quit draining from the abdomain.

The blood test man just got another sample so I guess I will be getting more blood. well I guess that is the account of me.

I surly appercieate the wonderfull job you done for me a the 11th field I hope you are happy at your new station Your pat. Stigers

Case 288

times. She was always very interested in a boy in the 141 Infantry and last time I saw her they had all plans set for their wedding. Just 10 days before the date they had selected for their marriage he was killed—when I hear things like that I stop complaining about my lot.

Our little flurry of work dropped off again and at this point I've taken up wood carving—very interesting.

Having early spring weather now and where the snow and cold were making things difficult last week, the mud and rain are doing it now.

Wednesday, February 7, 1945

No work during the night so I took off to Saarburg in the 2½ [two-and-a-half ton truck] this a.m. The roads from here to there are really chewed up—a month ago they were good but now they're awful. Nine new 1st Aux teams in here today—they have more teams here now than we have. Rumor has it that the rest of their teams are going with the 15th Army, which is about to go into action next to the 9th Army. The 6th Aux is on the way from the States and will then take over the 15th Army with the 1st Aux all coming down here. Where does that put us—Italy?

Thursday, February 8, 1945

Called from headquarters this a.m. to tell us we were moving. Left after lunch for Sarralbe, where Major Kennedy's platoon of the 10th Field set up yesterday. Town is just eight miles south of Sarrbrucken and is five miles from the front. Building is a ramshackle old place but at least is a building. Two 1st Aux teams here—Major McComb and Major Roberts. I'm the only 2nd Aux team and am in charge—sort of. We're behind a new Division—the 63rd.

Monday, February 12, 1945

Did a belly this afternoon—a bloody one—French civilian. Still not much work. Raining all day to beat the band—the mud at the front must be awful—fortunately we're in a building where the weather can't get at you. Russians now 60 miles west of Breslau and turning north.

Tuesday, February 13, 1945

Other two teams working fairly regularly, but we seem to miss the busy periods. One of the new teams asked me for advice on one of the thoraco-abdominal cases he had yesterday—I told him what I thought and he immediately disagreed. Several hours later I saw him and his first words were "Damned if you wasn't right." They'll learn.

There's a barbed-wire enclosure down the road from us—used by the Jerries for holding American officers. A small place—no beds—just straw on the floor—nothing like P.O.W.s in the States.

Wednesday, February 14, 1945

Hitched into headquarters this a.m.—it's a two-hour haul from here—but it was a beautiful day. The roads are terrible, however. Muddy ruts and completely broken in places. Numerous engineer groups are trying to keep them in repair. Sully fears that our outfit might make the Pacific—just the thought of it almost kills me. In the conversation he said I'd get my majority before I go home. Back here in one hitch to find some mail from Marion waiting for me—oh, how I love that gal!!

Thursday, February 15, 1945

XV Corps jumped off at dawn and so we're busy again. Just as they attacked, Jerry counterattacked—as per usual. It's 2 a.m. (16th Feb.) and I'm just getting to bed. Did four cases—three of them bellies and tough ones.

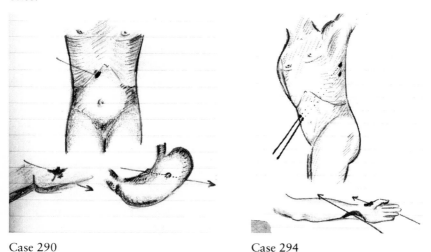

Case 290   Case 294

One guy had 14 perforations of small bowel plus a million other things—he'll probably die.

Had one Jerry in—18 years old but looked much younger. He was part of a division of others his age that just came here from the Russian front. He told how they were guarded by S.S. men and that how when the opportunity arose they not infrequently shot the guards.

Friday, February 16, 1945

Up for breakfast even though to bed late. The influx slowed up—three cases in all day. We did one this evening—a belly plus a lot of extremity wounds. Heard this evening that they're attacking again tomorrow morning so we'll probably be rushed again. They gained ground yesterday and today are in Hausweiller, Germany. Radio put out news of a big carrier task force (1,500 planes) raiding Japan.

Saturday, February 17, 1945

2 a.m. and just getting to bed—worked since just after breakfast this a.m. and I'm bushed. Did only three cases but had another die suddenly as he was being inducted—did a post immediately and he had what G. used to call the bad disease.

Supposedly this is only a local action—other parts of 7th Army not busy, but we certainly are. Getting some good cases and so far we're having awfully good luck.

Sunday, February 18, 1945

I'm convinced that Jerries are about the toughest human beings that God ever made 'cause they can take a lot of injury and still get by. Did a fellow tonight that certainly should die, but he got off the table in fine style and shows every indication that he's gonna live [case 300]. Brownie [Freeman Brown, anesthetist] gets about five bottles running and has so many tubes running in the guy that he looks like a "switchboard."

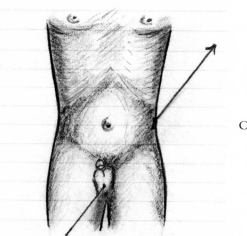

Case 300

Monday, February 19, 1945

I don't know whether or not it's my imagination or not, but the wounds I'm getting seem to be much worse. Had a fellow tonight that was shot in the right buttock; it then went anterior and to the left, coming out the left upper quadrant. It actually didn't do as much damage as you'd think, but it did enough. Work not heavy now but I'm still catching the heavy end of it—and being awfully lucky. They're making progress ahead of us here and there's some talk of moving.

Mail and packages today—some mail from October.

Tuesday, February 20, 1945

It seems that nobody else around here can catch a case but our team. Had another one of those from front to rear and side to side wounds tonight [case 302]. Fellow was a captain and before the operation he asked me to do all I could 'cause he had a lot of homework to take care of—a wife and three kids. He was "frapped up" proper and although he took the procedure well, I don't think he'll ever get back to his homework.

> Case 302. Gen'l condition on admission poor. Evidence of severe
> blood loss. B.P. 90/60
> P. 120. Abd. rigid and tender ++++. Urine 35 r.b.c. per./H.p.f.
> Diagnosis: G.S.W. perf. left buttock—right right upper quadrant
>   sv with F.C.C. ilium left severe. Secondary shock severe.
> Feb 28: Silver Star Awarded; Mar 3: Evacuated.

Wednesday, February 21, 1945

Changed shifts today so maybe somebody else will catch a little of this work. We have 25 patients here now and half of them are mine—and they are all bellies or thoraco-abdominals—real rough ones. So far we've been lucky and haven't lost a patient, but our luck can't last. There's an attack on tonight so we may get rooted out yet. Saarbrucken is the next point of interest.

Weather perfect—beautiful tonight and bombers have been going over all evening.

Thursday, February 22, 1945

Sully dropped in here this morning and made rounds with us—all our cases were doing OK and he was pleased with things in general, which is a help 'cause I'm more or less in charge. He said he's gonna send Brott, Brown, and me to Paris next week for a couple days—Paris!!

Saturday, February 24, 1945

There was a fairly strong Jerry counterattack this morning, and we know it here. I've done two cases and there's a shock ward still full so it's an all-night session for us. These two first aux teams are too slow and don't put out the work.

Sunday, February 25, 1945

Worked all last night and finally finished at breakfast time this morning. We did four cases—all tough ones—while the other two teams did one apiece—too slow. Slept all day and got up just in time for supper. They brought three little boys in here this evening—all with very severe wounds of their legs—one kid died and the other two will lose a leg or two. They were playing with a hand grenade. I'm thankful that my family is so far away from this war.

Monday, February 26, 1945

Our little spurt of activity quieted down again. Did a couple cases today but that's all. Unfortunately, one came in late and so it's now 3 a.m. and I'm just getting to bed. There's a move being planned which will take us rather close to the war again—Saareguemines, which is just this side of the border.

Wednesday, February 28, 1945

Worked until after breakfast this a.m. Had a fellow with a hip disarticulation and an arm amputation [case 309]. He pulled the pin of a hand grenade accidently while it was in his pocket. He was one mess.

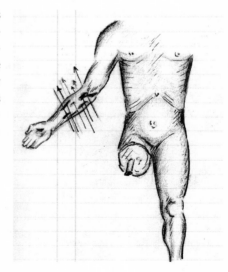

Case 309

Thursday, March 1, 1945

Saw a pretty good movie tonight and I really enjoyed it. It's so seldom that you see anything worthwhile. Learned at headquarters that we're definitely going to Paris on March 5 so that's something to look forward to. There's a belly case in now and we go on first call at midnight so I will be working for a while. Norquist, a 1st Aux orthopedic surgeon, left here today and I inherited a case from him that's a daisy—a bilateral amputation and both stumps are badly infected.

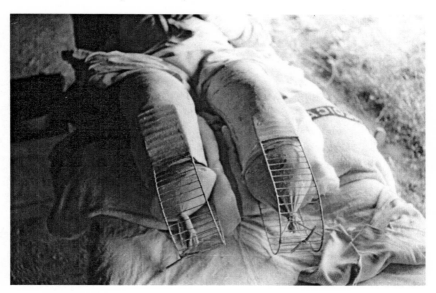

Bilateral amputation

Friday, March 2, 1945

Worked 'til breakfast time then spent all morning doing ward work so I'm tired now. Had a right nephrectomy during the night, which was a son of a gun. After that we had to incise and drain that bilateral amputation. He was a pretty foul mess.

Saturday, March 3, 1945

There's a push on and cases are piling in. We're on second call at midnight, which means that we'll be working all night.

Got a dandy new surgical book from Gordon today—as a Xmas present. Orr's *Operative Surgery*. It's an excellent new book and will be a big help. Got paid today and also got my whiskey ration—all set for Paris now.

Sunday, March 4, 1945

As per usual we got caught on another all-night job—worked thru until 11 a.m. and the platoon, except for a holding company, moved out from under us. Berget Blocksom's team replaced us and we're back at headquarters (Saarburg) all set to leave for Paris in the morning. We have 48 hours there—and a day coming and going.

Monday, March 5, 1945

Paris

My first night in Paris. We left Saarburg at 8 this morning and arrived here at 4:30 this afternoon. Had a freezing ride in an open weapons carrier and I was numb when we pulled in. Paris is a big city and looks much like New York to me. Lots of uniforms of all kinds but it doesn't spell too much of war on the surface. After being out in the sticks for so long it's good to get into a city once again. We're staying at the Alma—a small little hotel on Rue Montaigne, but we're eating at a nice place—the Mayflower Club on Rue Francois—very nice. Had supper there then took the "Metro" to the Folies B. [Folies Bergère]—quite a show with a gracious display of rather well-formed fronts—not half as suggestive as our shows at home.

After the show we were approached by three or four floozies but we went to the Red Cross Club on Place d'Concord and had doughnuts instead.

Tuesday, March 6, 1945

Paris

Slept like a log and almost missed breakfast—did all the P.X.s and bought a few items I needed, including a new E.T.O. [European theater of operations] jacket,[11] which is the latest item. Had lunch and then went downtown on the "Metro"—bought a bottle of perfume, then back to the Mayflower Club to get in on the 3:00 tour of the city. It just hit the high spots but it was good—and besides I don't like organized tours—saw the Arc de Triumph with its embossing flame, the Trocadero, Eiffel Tower, Notre Dame, the Latin Quarter, Napoleon's tomb, and other spots. Saw a British show this evening—Sir Cecil Hardwicke in *Yellow Sand*—it was very good.

We started out for a nightclub but the place was closed, so we wound up at the Red Cross and again had coffee and doughnuts. My aching dogs are killing me—so to bed.

Wednesday, March 7, 1945

Paris

Our last day in Paris and it was a full one. Started walking after breakfast and headed for the Latin Quarter down on the Left Bank below the cathedral—looked all around there—tried to find some watercolors but couldn't.

At noon, we shuffled around on the "Metro" and made our way over to the casino to get tickets, then back to the Mayflower Club for lunch.

After we ate, Brownie and I started walking again down in the shopping district. I did want to buy something, but the prices of everything were outrageous and even the simplest things were ridiculously priced. Paris had some beautiful stores and what merchandise I saw seemed to be good. Had a couple cocktails before supper and afterwards went to the Casino de Paris—what a show—more nudity than you'd see in the most crowded of shower rooms—but the thing was well done. Scenes and costumes were really beautiful and I enjoyed it. I must come back here with Marion sometime after the war—she'd love it. Coffee and doughnuts again at the Red Cross and then back here. We leave right after breakfast for Saarburg—and the "salt mines."

Thursday, March 8, 1945

Didn't get away from Paris 'til late and we were only 25 miles outside of the city by noon so we stopped and had lunch at the 1st Aux headquarters. Dinner with the 57th Field Hospital in Toul. They have 350 Russians—they had been P.O.W.s and were just liberated. Back in Saarburg by 8:30—tired out.

Friday, March 9, 1945

Up this morning early. Major Sullivan and Colonel Forsee out visiting the field hospitals so we didn't see them. Got orders to relieve Blocksom at Major Kennedy's platoon and got here in time for lunch. Lousy setup in an old, shelled-out monastery just short of Sarreguemines.

Lots of artillery and very little work. Looks like we're back in the war.

Saturday, March 10, 1945

One case in here all day and I caught it—fellow had his stomach just laid open from the pylorus to the cardia and presented quite a problem. Got him hooked together and off the table—now we'll see what happens.

This is a noisy place—for the first time in a long while we're back with the artillery and some of it was Jerry's. I slept, but it was a fitful sleep. I never will get used to that stuff, no matter how long this war lasts.

Sunday, March 11, 1945

Colonel Forsee here today with Sully. Had little to say, as per usual—is fat and just as lifeless as ever.[12] Told me that he understood I was doing a wonderful job and that when a promotion was available I'd get one— now we'll see how long it will take. My stomach case is doing very well and I'm encouraged. We're moving tomorrow—and I've been here only three days. Dive-bombers struck at something just over the hill today— what a noise!!

Monday, March 12, 1945

Moved this afternoon to the civilian hospital in Sarreguemines—only five miles but a more comfortable place in which to work. We have the second and third floors—quite a haul for the equipment.

There's a war going on 'cause from our window we can see occasional machine-gun tracers streaming off in various directions—and there's a 240-mm howitzer just off to our left that virtually shakes the building quite often. The German border is just about three miles or less ahead of us.

Wednesday, March 14, 1945

Another beautiful and sunny day—still no work but tomorrow the 7th Army attack starts at dawn. Directly to the north tonight at a distance

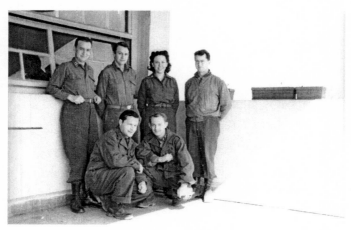

General
Surgical
Team 26,
March 1945

of 20 miles our bombers were met with a terrific amount of flak. It was a beautiful sight to see—fireworks at Rocky Glen. I tried to take a time exposure of it—so we'll see what I got.

Brott walked over the bridge into Germany today. I must do it tomorrow.

Thursday, March 15, 1945

At 1 a.m. I was blasted out of a sound sleep by the most terrific noise I've ever heard. Artillery all around the town and up and down to our right and left let loose. Searchlights were turned on and pointed upward in the direction of the attack, supposedly to create an artificial moonlight.

It continued for over an hour and must have been hell for Jerry. We had a perfect grandstand seat for the whole show. Casualties started coming in this a.m. and I've been working all day—it's now 3 a.m. of tomorrow and I'm bushed. One fortunate thing—we're getting lots of Jerries—and two cases that had been done today had recent operation wounds. One actually hadn't healed as yet. So you see Jerry is hurting.

Friday, March 16, 1945

To bed at midnight but there's a case in shock which will be ready soon. Up at 8 this morning, so I'm kinda tired right now. Work is coming in pretty heavy and we're all busy. Should have more teams but there just aren't any more.

Making some progress and they must be giving Jerry some hell seeing all the Jerry casualties we're getting.

Saturday, March 17, 1945

It's midnight and we've been working since 4 p.m. Got four hours' sleep this morning, which isn't enough, and we don't go off call 'til 8 in the morning. We're evacuating a good share of the cases unoperated because we simply can't do them all. Roberts is beaten to a pulp and McComb does too much work with his mouth. And as always we catch the load.

Sunday, March 18, 1945

Worked 'til 7 this morning—did some ward work and then to bed until 2 p.m. We had some rough cases during the night. One fellow got hit with an arsenal, from the looks of his back [case 323].

Had one fellow shot in the right hip and the slug ended up in his right heart. He died on the table, needless to say. Work has slowed up and I'm beginning to get hope of going thru the night. Pleased by simple things—a night's sleep.

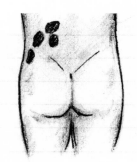

Monday, March 19, 1945

The pressure is definitely off and the resistance is practically nil, according to all reports. We had one case but that one was three in one [case 327].

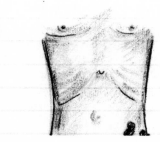

Case 323

Case 327. Diagnosis: GSW perf left lumbar region. Wd of exit at left costochondral junction in anterior axillary line. FCC ilium left. FC cartilage.

Evacuated 24 Mar.

News tonight has General Patton's army swinging down the Rhine behind the troops we're facing and now they have to turn and run to get out.

Tuesday, March 20, 1945

In bed at 4:30. This night shift is killing—we're only catching one case but it ruins the night completely. There's some talk of moving from here to join the 64th Field—a new outfit. Always a difficult task and something to make life more difficult—in an already difficult situation.

Wednesday, March 21, 1945

There's a case in now—a Jerry with a traumatic leg amputation that we'll be ready to do along about 1 a.m. He was injured yesterday and to stop the bleeding he tied a copper wire around his thigh just above the knee—his leg's a mess.

News is good tonight—there's very little organized resistance left in this pocket of the Rhine basin and prisoners are being taken in wholesale lots. This afternoon we walked over the hill to the temporary prison stockade and they had 800 in there—over 2,000 passed thru during the day.

Quite a few officers—one old fellow looked to be at least 65. Took pictures, of course.

Thursday, March 22, 1945

Got in bed at 3:30 this a.m. so I'm tired tonight. Patients all doing fairly well—lost only one at this stand so far—one out of 17, which is pretty good. Soon I'll probably hit a string of deaths.

5

Germany, the End of the War, and the Journey Home

Friday, March 23, 1945

No new cases—we change shifts today and we get the day shift, which is good. I can't get any real sleep in the daytime. Walked down to the bridge over the Saar today and took some pictures, then went on over into Germany.

The little town just on the other side of the river is badly torn up. Talked with a C.I.C. [Counter Intelligence Corps] officer today who was in Sarrbrucken when it fell—or just after—and he said the G.I.s went wild—put people out of their homes, looted places, and destroyed property and just had a wild destructive time. Germany, I'm afraid, is going to take a terrible physical beating. We're up for a move very shortly. The 3rd Unit went 80 miles into Germany yesterday.

Saturday, March 24, 1945

Always in the spring there's a questionable job to be done. Got word today we're going to Bad Durheim to stage—just for what, isn't told. But the 7th Army is about to go across the Rhine and I imagine we'll be over fairly early. The British, Canadians, and American 9th Army crossed the Rhine at Wessel on the lower Rhine and Patton's 3rd Army crossed near Oppenheim. There's great enthusiasm here about the war ending soon, but Germany is a big place.

Sunday, March 25, 1945, Palm Sunday

Checked out all our patients this morning—all of mine were in good shape except two—didn't lose a post-op patient at this stand and did 17 cases.

We're moving out of here at 4:30 tomorrow morning to go to Kaiserslautern to stage for the Rhine crossing.

Monday, March 26, 1945

Germany

Up at 4 this morning but we didn't get away as planned. Left Sarre-guemines at 6 a.m. and crossed the border, the Saar River, into Germany shortly after 6. Had a 60-mile ride to Kaiserslautern and in spite of heavy traffic got in before 11:00. Went thru Einoril and Hamburg. With few exceptions, every town we passed thru was pretty well destroyed. Not just an occasional house knocked down, but everything completely flat-tened. Didn't see very many people around. Once in a while a man with a small cart would be seen trying to salvage a few unbroken shingles from a mass of rubble. It seems to be the wish of everyone I know and of every-one I hear talk that we should completely destroy everything we come across and from the looks of things that is the main theme of the infantry. Everyone is taking particular delight in seeing such complete destruction here on German soil as we saw earlier in Africa, Sicily, Italy, and France. It seems that this in some small way is the beginning of payment of the great debt to the world the Germans owe.

We're set up at the 10th Field headquarters just outside of Kaiser-slautern—almost had to move shortly after we got here, but that was postponed. There's a staging area about 15 miles from here and that's where we're supposed to be—why we can't stage here is a mystery, but it's also the army.

Wednesday, March 28, 1945

Up at 6 a.m. but didn't get away until after 10, always waiting on trans-portation. Stopped at the 10th Field headquarters at Monsheim. Had lunch there and waited 'til 2:00 for clearance to go over the bridge. We passed thru Worms at 3 p.m.—it was beaten up something awful—in parts was just nothing but piles of brick and plaster.

The bridge there was blown by the Jerries and a heavy pontoon bridge was up. A red and white sign with three large stars and bearing the title "The Alexander Patch Bridge to Germany" denoted the bridge's name. The Rhine here wasn't very large but in peacetime must have been a beautiful river. The land on each side is quite flat but 10 miles or so to the north and south the hills start and rise sharply. I took lots of pictures in Worms and crossing the bridge but all from a moving vehicle.

Too, there was heavy smoke around the river (two bridges upstream had been knocked out yesterday). We are set up in a dirty, filthy school building and why we didn't set up in tents is a mystery to everybody.

This clearing company (119th) is new. This town we're in, Lampertheim, wasn't damaged too badly but didn't escape completely.

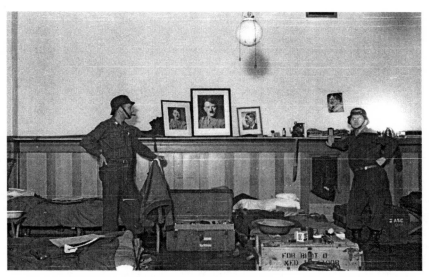

Set up in a school at Lampertheim: "Paul Samson [thoracic surgeon], Hitler, and myself"

Friday, March 30, 1945

Just finished a case—a boy from Wilkes Barre—he was in rough shape when he came in and still is—I'm afraid he's gonna die.

Only one case in here all day—the 44th is out of the line—replaced by the 63rd—and the clearing station is moving tomorrow so what will happen to us I don't know. Beatty's and Plyler's platoons are away ahead of us but in another direction. We seem to be heading southeast toward Heidelberg. We heard that it had been declared an open city by Jerry and then when our boys went in Jerry shelled it. Consequently the G.I.s pulled back and started to pound it with artillery. That's what happened at Mannheim—it's now just a pile of broken bricks.

Saturday, March 31, 1945, Mom's and Ruth's birthday

Up at 0530 hours. Patient I did last night developed pulmonary edema and died—not good but he never was any rose [case 332].

The clearing station moved out today so business will be nil 'til we move again—which is all right with me. I've never been so fed up or sick

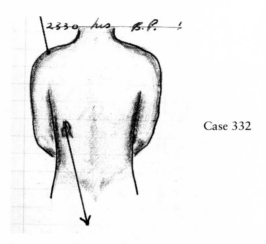

Case 332

of anything in all my life. Tomorrow I start my 30th month overseas—too long. Ruthie is 19 months old and still I haven't seen her.

April 1, 1945, Easter Sunday

And the Easter parade this year is through Germany. There aren't many countries left so maybe I'll be spending an Easter at home next year. Not even Mass—can't go to German churches. No chaplain here—none all this week so not a very holy Easter week. The 44th Division is going in on the left of the 45th Division—between 45th and 3rd Army in a few days so our inactive status may be cut short. There's been considerable rape and looting going on in this town so it's been placed off limits—now we can't go outside this building—very dull existence.

Tuesday, April 3, 1945

Got away after lunch and headed northeast for the 120th Medics just south of Aschaffenburg. That's the town where a German major got the townspeople all hot and bothered—had them sniping and throwing grenades—the 45th just pulled back and for four days just blasted the town—dive-bombers kept working it over 'til now there's nothing left but smoldering ruins. Madman Colonel Ross took three of our trucks away this evening to help move Plyler in the morning. That means that we're going to have to wait here tomorrow while the rest of the trucks go ahead, unload, and come back.

Rather a pleasant wait here tonight, however—this platoon was with the 45th when they got into the Jerry liquor warehouse. I've never seen such a supply of cognac and stuff in all my life. Benedictine, brandy, etc.—all the best there is. They were generous and gave us a good ration.

Thursday, April 5, 1945

Rooted out of bed at midnight—told to pack and off we started on a blackout 50-mile ride. Rode all night, getting to our area near Mernes at 5:30. I thought surely we were going right on thru to the Jerry side of things and we easily could have—got lost several times as it was. We're back with the 45th Division and they're moving very rapidly now. Just a little too fast. We're all set up here but we're going out again tomorrow another 50 miles or so. Did two cases—one a little Bessarabian girl with an amputation of her leg—15 years old and has been here in Germany working a period of servitude for the past five years.

We're in the province of Bavaria now—it's a profoundly Catholic state and it was here that there was a great suppression of the church—even an attempt to make German the official language of the Mass. These people are anti-Nazi and have a difficult time understanding our nonfraternization program. My friend Father Carney has met several priests here who speak good English and they have tried to be friendly with him. He's had a difficult time of it trying to make them understand.

Friday, April 6, 1945

Been waiting all afternoon for transportation—just got word we're not moving until tomorrow morning. Tore down most everything this morning after evacuating our patients. McComb had a death on the table last night and two died in shock. (Had total of eight cases here and five died—none of ours.) We never pack our personal things until the truck is at our door and ready to go—there are always too many changes to do otherwise. Cold and raining here tonight.

Saturday, April 7, 1945

Most all the hospital moved out this morning and because there was a possibility the trucks wouldn't get back to us tonight, my team came up on the last ambulance—nothing but musette bags. We traveled about 50 miles northeast and now we're halfway from Sarreguemines to Berlin. Just outside the town of Hausen, a little northeast of Ostheim. About 20 miles below here we were held up for three hours because Jerries had come back in a town thru which we had to pass. We're sorta getting out on a limb. The clearing station is actually 20 miles behind us and is coming up tonight; the battalion aid of the 180th Infantry is just down the road—behind us. It's 10:00 now and we're all set to go.

Saw some T.D.s [tank destroyers] go by here before dark and one was funny—sticking out of the turret was a fellow wearing goggles and a high silk hat!

We're moving fairly fast now, just as fast as the "impedimenta" of war will allow. Jerry isn't very far—this afternoon while we were waiting for clearance a good ways down the road, a G.I. came walking across the field with three Krauts whom he had found in the hills just behind that station. There's no organized resistance—just an occasional firefight. No artillery at all.

Methinks this war is coming to an end.

Monday, April 9, 1945

The past 24 hours have been sort of a tough deal. We got in 11 cases last night at midnight just as I came on call. Of the group, we were able to evacuate five but the other six took all evening to do and we were scheduled to move at 8:30 a.m. Before the last case was done the place was torn down except for a small holding company. I was tired but we had to pack and get ready—we had done half of the six cases—the other two teams did the remaining three. At this point we're moving in ducks (DUKW's)[1] and they ride much better than trucks but don't hold as much and are very difficult to load—so high from the ground.

Moved about 50 miles to a place just east of Konigshofen. I must

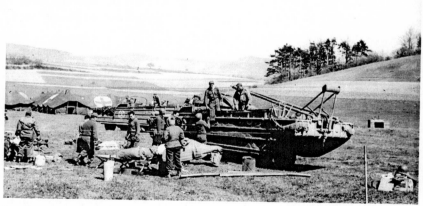

Loading a DUKW

repeat once again that Germany is certainly a beautiful country—at least this part of it is. The weather is perfect now—warm and clear—and the sky is full of planes. The part of Germany we're heading for must be taking a terrible beating now.

Tuesday, April 10, 1945

We can't get a good night's sleep no matter how hard we try—got rooted out of bed at midnight and worked 'til 3. It seems that all we're getting are Jerries and they're pretty well shot up.

Wednesday, April 11, 1945

A red-letter day. I captured a Kraut and all by my lonesome. Drove down to the holding unit some 25 miles in our rear to see the three patients I left—they're all OK. While there and just as we were leaving, a German civilian came hurrying across the fields waving a white flag. He was all excited and when he quieted down we (a Jerry plane just now dove on the road alongside of us and strafed a long column of vehicles—I dashed out but saw only the tail end of the firing. The whole column opened up on him—but missed) learned that his daughter had been wounded by a booby trap set on a door in the military barracks just up the hill from our last area. Three days before we rummaged all thru that place but fortunately missed that door. We drove over to his place and to his home. Although the outside had the customary pile of "horseshit" in front, the inside was spic-and-span. The gal wasn't hurt too badly—at least she wasn't (that plane just came back again but I didn't get out in time to see the firing) a field hospital case. They were very appreciative and gave us a dozen eggs in payment.

On the way home as we left the town of Oberelsbach, a Jerry soldier stepped out in the road with his hands up in the air—a tough-looking nut but he appeared scared to death. We took him aboard the weapons carrier and I frisked him but all he was carrying was a loaf of bread and a piece of baloney. He lived in Worms. 'Cause nobody would believe us we got him out of the car and took pictures.

After driving another half hour we met up with a convoy of trucks carrying Jerries, so we just turned him over to the M.P.s and got credit for the capture of one Jerry.

Friday, April 13, 1945

From London this morning we heard the sad news of the president's death—yesterday afternoon at Warm Springs. I really felt sick when I heard it—I can't help but feel that we have lost a great man at a time when we most needed him. History will rightfully give him a place among America's—among the world's—immortals.

Evacuated all our patients today—supposedly we're moving in the a.m. I drove down to the holding company and got rid of my three patients there—they were all doing quite well. Weather continues sunny and warm.

Saturday, April 14, 1945

No move today but we're all torn down ready to go. Tomorrow supposedly. Played a ball game this afternoon and then a couple of volleyball games—I feel stiff as a poker tonight but good.

I don't know how to write down in words just how I feel right now but I'd like to try—this once. It's 11:00—the lights have been turned off and I'm writing this by candles. Brown and Brott are in bed—one reading by candlelight—the other by flashlight. The stove is still on and it's puffing away like a tired veteran. Brown and I started about 7:00 to have a few drinks while we were writing our daily letters—on thru the 9:00 news we drank—past some 10:00 program—and now it's 11:00. McComb the windbag; Roberts the undecided; and a few lesser lights have been in and gone—and here I am. Just a little stewed—and into bed I'll get—when all the time I'd like to fly thru time and space to you, Marion, to be with you—to lay with you—to love you. I must soon be with you—I love you so.

Tuesday, April 17, 1945

Trucks came just before noon. Packed and away by 2 p.m. heading for Plyler's platoon and from there on to join the 120th Medics at Lauf directly east of Nuremberg. A dirty, dusty ride in the back of an open weapons carrier. In some towns a few people wave and smile and always the children wave and act glad to see you.

But mostly people just stare. As we came near Lauf, some towns were still burning. Saw an old man and woman searching through the burning embers of what yesterday was probably their home.

As we came into Lauf, five Jerry jet-propelled planes came racing across the sky. Ack-ack from all directions went pointing at them but that's all it did.

Set up in the dark—the clearing station was holding four cases for us but we were able to get rid of two. It's midnight and I'm going to bed for a while—'til a case is ready.

Wednesday, April 18, 1945

What a night. Discovered that we were right in the center of one hell of a lot of artillery and they blasted all night but we worked all night—at least 'til 5 this morning. Had three air raids during the night and what a racket—we got back in the war awful sudden like. We were on call 'til 4 p.m.

Had a couple air raids this afternoon—a bomb was dropped in Lauf and we got a case hit by same bomb—that's getting awfully close. Nuremberg is half occupied now—the 3rd and 45th have it surrounded and word has it that they'll take it tomorrow.

Sunday, April 22, 1945

I've neglected everything for the past few days because I've had time for nothing but work and sleep, and not much sleep at that. In three days we did 16 cases and they were rough ones at that. We've had more air raids—I've heard more artillery—just more war generally speaking than I've seen in some time—and all too damn close. We're near a little town called Lauf—it's five miles out of Nuremberg on the highway running east and we were here much before Nuremberg was taken. Lauf was a center of a lot of equipment, supplies, and troops, and the Jerries knew it and they bombed it frequently—we'd get patients just a few minutes after they were hurt—again, much too close.

We've done just about half the work here—16 out of 36 cases and there were two other teams working with us and two additional teams took a night's stand each. There's been hell to pay about one of the teams—McComb's—he's been called for stalling, ducking work, being too slow, etc., and so he's being shipped out of here soon.

Nuremberg finally fell yesterday and so except for a little work from the 14th Armored, this stand has spent itself. We've got some sick turkeys, too. I must get into town and get some pictures—there's a sports *platz* in town where many Nazi ceremonies were held—there's an American flag flying there today.

Monday, April 23, 1945

The clearing station moved out today so we're just about closed. Plyler's platoon has jumped us and is some 40 miles south of here. We've got such a load now that we'll have to sit here for a few days 'til we can transport our cases. We're actually in 3rd Army area and no 7th Army evacs will come near us. Now I suppose we won't be able to evacuate to a 3rd Army hospital.

I did a patient named K. when the rush first started—a mild little fellow with lots of small gut all shot up—next to him in the ward is a Jerry—and it so happens that this particular Jerry is the one who shot K.—a nice fellow to have on your left.

Tuesday, April 24, 1945

The rain has finally stopped and again the sun is out—so much nicer in tents in the sun. All my patients doing OK with one exception, and he doesn't look too good [expired fifth post-operative day]. Nothing new coming in here now. Had a Jerry plane over here earlier this evening and he got a hot reception with ack-ack—but they never hit anything.

Wednesday, April 25, 1945

Had a death today—a boy that should never have died except for trouble he previously had. I mean to say his belly wound alone was doing nicely but nevertheless he's dead.

Drove into Nuremberg this afternoon for a look—it's a total and complete loss. A large city—population 400,000 in prewar days, and now it's leveled. Just where these people will start is a mystery to me—I must say our destruction is thorough.

Saturday, April 28, 1945

Little of anything to report for the past three days. Evacuated all our cases today to a 3rd Army evac just north of Erlangen. I rode up with a load of my sicker ones. We're making a jump of over 100 miles our next trip and it will probably be tomorrow. I'm very much afraid that we'll get in on the battle for Munich 'cause 7th Army is just about 35 miles from there now.

Russians and 1st Army met on the Elbe yesterday, April 27th.

Reuters claims Himmler offered unconditional surrender to British and U.S. if Russia would be left out—was turned down.

Wednesday, May 2, 1945

Lohhof

Trucks came for us yesterday morning and we left our area at Lauf just after lunch. A cold long ride in an open weapons carrier—and it snowed all the way on the 1st of May. Stopped off at 10th Field head-quarters and picked up some mail—then on to Pilot's platoon—and the ride got colder. They had been fired on that morning from the woods behind them by small-arms fire. Left there just before dark and rode till

11 p.m. I was wet and cold and we had to pitch tents in the black and wet and cold. Got in bed finally at 3:30 a.m.

We're eight miles from Munich, just north of it—Dachau, a concentration camp, was liberated the day before yesterday. I went through it today. I've read much about the horrors and atrocities of such places and was always, as with everyone, much in doubt as to the truth of such things—but today I saw it all. A crematory with four ovens and several adjoining rooms piled high with naked, starved, horrible-looking bodies.

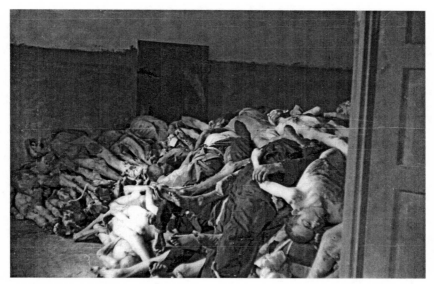

Dachau, May 2, 1945

A gas chamber built to resemble a shower room in which the victims unknowingly washed themselves to death. 10 men a month from each of the prison's blocks were cremated—the men volunteered and were glad to—to get away from the place.

I walked thru the prison proper with a Jugoslav who had been there 50 months. The S.S. guards were still lying around the outer fence where they were shot down in their tracks by Yanks.

Some had fallen into the small moat that surrounded the wire enclosure, and up through the few feet of shivering clear water they stared and saw nothing.

32,000 prisoners were held there and there was room for only a

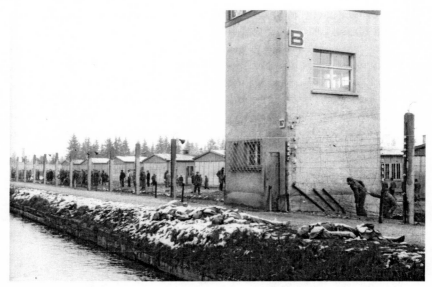

Dead guards in the snow at Dachau.

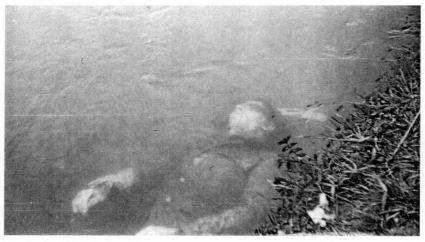

The body of an SS guard in a canal.

small part of that number. Triple and sometimes beds to the depth of six and then two and three in each bed. I walked in one barracks room and a French almost-starved Jew whined, "American" and put his fingers to his mouth as if to beg for food. I felt guilty 'cause I didn't have any to give him. I never saw a human look so bad and yet be alive.

[The liberation of the concentration camp at Dachau will be for-ever colored by the acts of some of the liberators. While some details remain in dispute, there can be no doubt that American soldiers—perhaps unhinged by the unexpected horrors they witnessed in the camp on top of weeks of nonstop combat—shot and killed unarmed German soldiers, most of them from the SS, as they attempted to surrender. This included wounded soldiers who had been sent to Dachau to recover from injuries incurred on the battlefields of the Ostfront. Anthony Beevor asserts, "More than 500 SS guards were killed, some by the prisoners, but most by American troops sickened by what they saw in the camp."[2]

The subsequent investigation by the Seventh Army inspector general concluded that the facts justified court-martial for a number of individu-als on charges of murder, but ultimately no trials were held and no pun-ishment meted out. As Rick Atkinson wrote: "Here surely was victor's justice, tinged with the sour smell of sanctimony, a reminder that honor and dishonor often traveled in trace across a battlefield, and that even a liberator could come home stained if not befouled."[3]]

All Germans in Italy surrendered unconditionally as of yesterday noon.

Thursday, May 3, 1945

Drove into Munich this morning just to have a look around and to find 45th Division signal repair. It snowed like the devil all the way in and was bitter cold. Munich appears very much like all these other bombed- and shelled-out towns—it's completely down—what remains of a few places is nothing but a shell of what they were. Things are such a complete mess that I can't understand how they'll ever be able to make a city out of the place again. There's going to be chaos in this country after this war.

News today tells of more surrendering. Hamburg yielded to the Brit-ish. Berlin fell last night.

I'm sure the rest will fall this week. The 45th Division was relieved today and there's talk we may go with another division.

Friday, Saturday, May 4 and 5, 1945

Did a case—a chest case—at 4 a.m. He was shot in the back in Munich by an M.P. when he failed to halt when challenged. Got word at break-fast time that we were gonna follow the 86th Division so we evacuated him to the 93rd. We're going to leave a holding company—Roberts had a sick patient but he died in time to change plans. Left Lohhof at 3:30, drove through Munich to Haag going like a bat out of hell. Had only four trucks so we only had the bare essentials of a field hospital—the kitchen and all other teams were left behind—supposedly they were to be shuttled up later in the day. We had orders to meet the clearing station of the 86th Division in Haag—we waited 'til 7:00 before they appeared.

We bummed a sandwich in a division kitchen there in town and except for that we were empty. The clearing station, we learned, was setting up in Kraiburg so we drove on to there. Division was there but the surgeon's office, the S3, the collecting company, and a battalion aid station there in town didn't know where the clearing station was. What a mixed-up mess. We finally bivouacked in a field in the rain. I must say I slept pretty well. A battalion aid station was set up in a Jerry house right next to us so I got Miss Lang a room there. This morning Lo Balbo the M.A.C. [Medical Administrative Corps] was supposed to bring back trucks, but he appeared at noon with nothing but some bread and jam and coffee—our first meal. The clearing station, we learned, had moved some 25 miles from Kraiburg so off we go again. Jerries all over the place walking in to towns along the road—in wagons, in vehicles, and some on horseback. All turning in and a sorry bunch they are.

Got in Mitter-Garching this afternoon at 4 p.m. and we're staying here tonight. We caught up with the clearing station—a queer bunch—just interested in how many guns and cameras they can find. They are set up in a Nazi school—Hitler Jugend. It was obviously quite a place in its day. They've already got orders to move to a concentration area in the morning to a place in Austria, so we haven't set up. Tonight we're sleeping in a civilian home across the street from the school. A small and modest place but very neat and clean. The people were Catholics. Had a son in the army and evidently he was killed.

The news is most encouraging and there are great reports—some have the war over, but at any rate it's ending quickly—and I'm happy it is.

Sunday, May 6, 1945

Still in Mitter-Garching. The clearing station moved out this morning but we're gonna stay here 'til they find a place where they're gonna settle down for a while. It's impossible to keep up with them with the few trucks we have.

All that's left of Germany's army is that part in Czechoslovakia—and the forces in Norway—it will probably be a few days before they surrender. The rest of the hospital caught up with us today so now we have a kitchen.

Monday, May 7, 1945

Germany surrendered unconditionally to the Allies this a.m. 0241 hours at Rheims, France. It was not yet officially announced by the Allies but will be tomorrow. Tomorrow has been designated as V-E day.

Still sitting here in Mitter-Garching doing nothing. Weather very nice now.

Tuesday, May 8, 1945

This afternoon at 3 p.m. it was announced by the Big Three that Germany had unconditionally surrendered to the Allies—the final deadline is to be 0001 hours, May 9, 1945. It's hard to believe and maybe more difficult to appreciate the fact that now at long last this war in Europe is finished—a war in which 20 million people lost their lives—and now there still remains the big job of doing away with the Japs. There is no question what their fate will be, but the price will be heavy and the time may be long. Drove down to Salzburg in Austria, then on 24 kilometers to Berchtesgaden—a pretty little town at the foot of the Austrian Alps. I never in my life saw such beautiful scenery. Sparkling green valleys preparing to spring into bloom, from which sharply rise high hills that reach into the clouds and beyond. Their tops wear a broken mantle of snow.

The hotel which has frequently but wrongly been shown as Hitler's home is situated halfway up the side of one of these mountains and must have been a beautiful spot. But now it's in ruins—bombed to nothing. I picked up a few glasses in the basement as souvenirs. Hitler's home is located right on the very top of this mountain—we drove almost to it but finally the heavy snow blocked the road, leaving an hour and a half climb on foot—but we didn't have time to make it. I took lot of pictures and kicked myself a thousand times because I didn't have Kodachrome.

Hitler picked the most beautiful spot in Germany to build his home—but now it's in ruins—just as his Nazi Party is in complete ruin!

Friday, May 11, 1945

Left Mitter-Garching just after lunch and drove over to 10th Field headquarters on the lake 30 miles northeast of Salzburg. When we got there we found out all teams were being called in the next day so we just took off for Augsburg. Stopped off at 5 p.m. for lunch—spam, eggs, and a quart of beer—tasted pretty good.

Drove up the autobahn and had a real good ride. Just south of Munich there's a stretch of the road which is perfectly flat and is at least

10 miles long. The Jerries had planes hidden in the trees alongside the road and used the highway as a runway. There were many planes and all kinds strung out along the road. I'm sure it never could be found from the air—it was never bombed.

Got lost in Munich but finally arrived at 2nd Aux at 9:30 p.m. Still light.

Saturday, May 12, 1945

Used most of the day turning in instruments, getting my laundry done, then played a ball game with the enlisted men. Had a pretty good party tonight—lots of scotch—all teams back but a few—so had a good time.

Monday, May 14, 1945

Life here seems to be one continuous party for some people and getting to sleep is therefore difficult. If I have to spend several months here I'll go completely nuts.

Played a ball game with the E.M. [enlisted men] tonight—with the short mess and this exercise I should lose weight.

Tuesday, May 15, 1945

Had a most enjoyable trip today into Austria and Italy—the latter briefly. Bob Wiley [Robert H. Wyley, general surgeon], Charlie Westerfield, Fred Burich [Fred T. Burich, assistant general surgeon], Todd Towery, and Brown and Brott. Down to Oberammergau, Garnisch-Partenkirchen, Innsbruck, Brenner Pass, then up along the Inn River then back to Parten-kirchen and home. I've never seen such beautiful scenery in all my life and, darling, I promise you right now I'm gonna bring you back here to see all this 'cause you'd enjoy it so. (I love you!)

The Olympics were held in Partenkirchen in 1936—saw the ski run and skating rink, etc.

There's a railroad there that runs to the top of a mountain—2,900 meters up, beautifully dressed in a snow-top dress. Innsbruck lies along the Inn River in a valley between two steep mountain ranges. Took the cable car there to the top of a peak 2,300 meters high.

The lift is made in two stages—it seems as if it goes right on up to heaven.

Went south then to the Brenner Pass and stepped into Italy just across the border. Took lots of pictures so you can see it all, darling. Got back at 11:30 tired and ready for bed.

Thursday, May 17, 1945

Waited around all day to go to the 11th Field but the guide they were supposed to send up never came so we're still waiting. Examined today for the service rating score—I've got 142 points and so I stand pretty high. Now I'll see how far it gets me.

[To determine when personnel were eligible to return to the United States, the army developed the service rating score. A soldier's score was calculated based on four criteria: one point for every month in service; one point for every month in service overseas; five points for every combat award (including battle stars); and twelve points for every dependent child under twelve.]

Friday, May 18, 1945

Left headquarters in Augsburg at 2 p.m. and headed northwest. Took the autobahn to Stuttgart—every cockeyed bridge on the thing had been blown out so there were numerous detours. Stuttgart is just another pile of rubble. Then up through Heilbrunn, which is also in ruins—and on up to a little town called Oberdielbach. Arrived about 10 p.m. 11th Field only partly set up but is ready for business. We're just 25 miles from Heidelberg.

Had a dusty, dirty, difficult ride up here. Sleeping in a ward tonight.

Saturday, May 19, 1945

We were on call all day and a lot of crud came in. This is not a very pleasant assignment, to say the least. The setup is nice but doing this type of work after doing nontransportable is trying, to say the least. We're to move in a day or so to Eberbach into a *Gasthaus* and the hospital into a school building.

Sunday, May 20, 1945

Moved into Eberbach today into a Gasthaus and school building. Quite a nice little town located on the Neckar River, 25 miles east of Heidelberg. The work is turning out to be nothing but piddling stuff and most boring.

Monday, May 21, 1945

Back to writing charts—we caught about 20 patients today but there's little to do for any of them except evacuate them to the rear. We can't operate on anything here that will require longer than five to seven days for recovery—which rules most everything out. Raining and quite cold.

Tuesday, May 22, 1945

A quiet day—rain, then sun, then more rain. Did a ruptured appendix tonight. A clearing station held the fellow since last midnight until this evening. Not good. He had a belly full of pus and will be lucky if he makes it.

Stars and Stripes printed a list of new battle stars today—we now get a total of nine. Which gives me 157 points—but now points won't mean anything for medical officers, I suppose.

Wednesday, May 23, 1945

Miss Levy bought mail back from headquarters this a.m. Got three letters from Marion—I don't know how I can possibly be more anxious than I have been to get home but I am—it seems that this period of waiting will never end.

Admissions have fallen off.

Thursday, May 24, 1945

My 24 hours off. Drove over to Heidelberg this afternoon and looked around—a very nice little town—85,000 in prewar days. Went through the university library. They have all the files and records of I.G. Farben and several other companies there now all catalogued for our use—patents, etc. Little or no damage in Heidelberg.

Heard today from the adjutant that we are being recalled in a few days—the 2nd Aux is going someplace and in all probability it's back to Italy—but I certainly hope it's home.

Sunday, May 27, 1945

To church this morning in the town church—they have a small number of pews set aside for the military—for we can't mingle with the people—the nonfertilization policy, as it's called in 1st Army.

A little work today but only a little—no word as yet about leaving, but I'm so sick of this place I could scream—I hope I'm not gonna be this restless the remainder of my life.

Saturday, June 2, 1945

Price brought back some mail from our headquarters, but I only got one letter from Marion. She and the kids had been to the circus in Madison Square Garden and they had a whirl. (When am I gonna get back in their lives?)

Monday, June 4, 1945

Just finished an appendix—that's the sixth one we've had in two weeks.

Heard a new rumor tonight—officers with 115 points are being sent home immediately—but it's just a rumor so far.

Thursday, June 7, 1945

Left after breakfast to come down here for a few days—have a Gasthaus on the Ammersee about 30 miles south of Augsburg. A big lake—several (three to four) miles wide and 11 miles long. We're at one end of it and at the other the Alps rise up to the sky—kinda pretty. Several sailboats, pretty good swimming—but the food is pretty scarce.

Friday, June 8, 1945

Sailed practically the whole day. This afternoon there was a good breeze up and we really ran along the water. Sun very hot and so I'm getting color in a hurry. Blocksum left the outfit today to become C.O. of the 11th Field—just a move to try and get home quicker.

Sunday, June 10, 1945

Orders came in today for our return to Italy—they have us routed by way of Marseilles—a trip of some 1,500 miles, when actually by going thru the Brenner Pass it's only 270 miles—but that's the way the army does things. Sully came back today with news of our Italian group. Says they're in a nice hotel on Lake Garda halfway between Venice and Milan—sometimes still out with F.H.s taking care of P.O.W.s. Says they're anxious to get us back. Party here for Blocksum and it's pretty drunk out.

Thursday, June 14, 1945

Left Augsburg at 0600 hours this a.m. and arrived here in Riva, Italy, at 2200 hours.

Down thru Oberammergau, Garnisch-Partenkirchen, Innsbruck, Brenner Pass, Bolzano, Trento, Revereto, and then to here. Riva is situated on Lake Garda, a beautiful body of water four to six miles wide, 30 some miles long. Around its sides sharp rocky mountains rise up suddenly. Headquarters is in a hotel—Albergo Lido—rather a nice place—some 60 rooms. Nice beach club next door for bathing. Colonel Forsee away but we're headed for lots of work on the records.

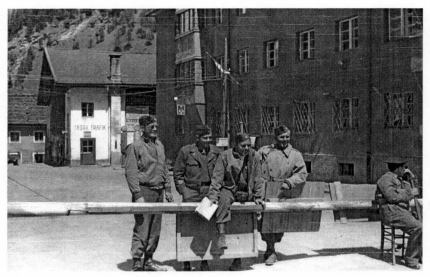

Second Aux officers at the Austria/Italy border, June 14, 1945.

Friday, June 15, 1945

Had a good night's sleep. Did little of anything but swim and get to see this place. Rode down to the Lake to 5th Army headquarters this afternoon along a road which is cut out of the rock. I think there are 70 tunnels along 25 miles. In the longest tunnels they set up lathes and presses, etc., and in this bombproof place turned out airplane engines—very clever.

Monday, June 18, 1945

Spent most of the day working on records. Gordon and I are collecting all the livers and it's quite a job. I worked all evening too 'cause tomorrow I'll be away all day—going to Venice for the day. Had my daily sunning at noon over at the A.R.C [American Red Cross].

No mail—it's been days now.

Wednesday, June 20, 1945

Working in the "gas chamber"—the record room—all day—what a lousy job it is—the records actually aren't worth a dime—but the colonel insists—a large report is all that matters to him.

[The "large report"—for which my father did all the charts and graphs and supplied the photographs—became *Forward Surgery of the Severely Wounded: A History of the Activities of the 2nd Auxiliary Surgical Group, 1942–45*. Produced in two volumes, it ran to 931 pages and described the clinical treatment of the various types of wounds the surgeons of the Second Aux encountered. It also detailed the administration and logistics of managing mobile surgical units under the most difficult of circumstances and gave the history of the operational activities of the unit. My father may have thought it "not worth a dime," but it was a priceless source of information for me. By the time I started this project in earnest, to my knowledge no Second Aux officer was still alive. As they toiled away in the Gas House, grumbling all the while, their assignment was to produce a report for the surgeon general, but I like to think they were unknowingly doing it for me as well, so that I could help to tell their story.]

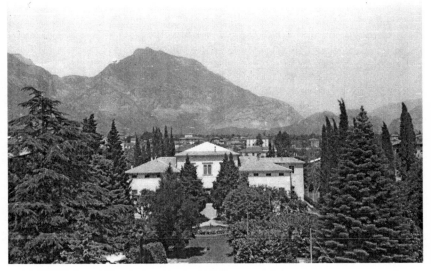

The "Gas House" at Riva, Italy, June 1945.

Thursday, June 21, 1945

Dance this evening at the Riva Hotel—a nice quiet affair and very much unlike a 2nd Aux party. The reason being the colonel stayed until the last dog was dead.

I'm being sent out tomorrow to Cortina to German hospital to help speed up evacuation of Jerry wounded—just going alone.

Friday, June 22, 1945

Cortina, Italy

Drove about 150 miles in a 2½ and arrived here in time for dinner. Thru Trento, Bolzano to here—we're just 30 miles south of the Austrian border. This is a garden spot if I ever saw one—a beautiful little Alpine village nestled down between peaks that reach some 10,000 feet into the sky.

There's still a little snow on their tops. There's swimming, horseback riding, and very little work to do, so I hope the job lasts a while.

Living in a most modern little villa and am very comfortable.

Sunday, June 24, 1945

Made rounds with Captain Shuppler [a German doctor] and the Jerry lieutenant colonel. They have some foul infections—about 88 cases left, but they're all crocks and it will be a few weeks before they can be moved. I don't mind 'cause I'd just as soon sit here as in Riva.

Shuppler, the orthopedic man, has written a paper on the marrow nailing of fractures.[4] I corrected his English version of it this evening. It's something entirely new and as yet is untried in the States.

Sunday, July 1, 1945

Left Cortina at 7:30 for Riva. Had lunch at 33rd Field with Tom Ballantine, then on to Riva—got here at 3 p.m. 14 nurses alerted to go home but no word about officers. Several more low-point men being transferred out. Saw a U.S.O. show tonight over at the Red Cross—just fair.

Monday, July 2, 1945

47 of our nurses got orders today—they're leaving for Naples in a few days to start the journey home. The latest dope on officers is that we're on the October sailing list—what a kick in the pants that is.

Tuesday, July 3, 1945

The crowning blow was struck this morning—at officers' call, Colonel F. announced we were in category 4 and he added that we were scheduled to go home in December—it just about floored everybody—I just can't believe that it means what it says. Nurses and enlisted men have already started to leave for home and in a few days almost all the nurses will be gone. I don't know what I'll tell Marion.

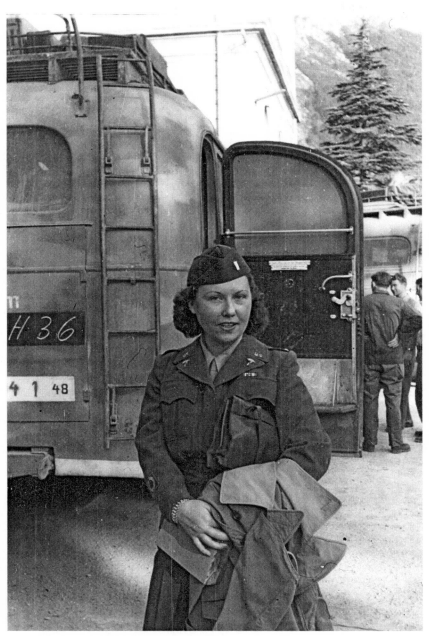

Nurses leaving for home, July 1945.

Wednesday, July 4, 1945

A quiet, sunny 4th of July; no excitement around here whatsoever and most everyone is feeling pretty blue about the proposed December trip.

Friday, July 6, 1945

All but seven of our nurses left this morning for Verona to fly to Naples. They're joining the 26th General Hospital there to go home with them—but we sit on, and as things stand now until December.

"Gas House" going full blast. I had to turn down a week at Lake Maggiore but I'm gonna have a week in Venice later.

Got our seventh battle star today—the Rhine crossing. We're supposed to get one for Anzio, too.

July 7 to 15, 1945

Just pure routine days in the Gas House—with little doing but graphs and swimming.

Wednesday, July 18, 1945

Left Garda Monday the 16th and drove to Venice—a city of 126 islands and 144 bridges—stayed at the Bella Riva. Walked and rode in a gondola all over the town. It's unique but it stinks.

The Lido is a beautiful place nearby and we enjoyed a day out there. Hitched back here in five rides this afternoon. Colonel back from Caserta with news that our sailing date would very likely be changed to September and that some high-point officers may go home sooner—good.

Saturday, July 28, 1945

Finished all my graphs today finally. I've worked morning, noon, and night to get them done. Going to Stressa in a.m. for five days. Lots of good rumors which have us going home in a few weeks or so.

Monday, August 6, 1945

Pappy Gay's [possibly Ellery C. Gay, maxillofacial surgeon] news still is the big order of the day. We're supposed to leave on the 10th. The colonel treats us like schoolchildren and it's like pulling teeth to get anything out of him. He's a poor excuse for a man.

The first atomic bomb fell on Japan yesterday and according to all reports it must have raised hell with them. There is talk of a desire for peace on the part of the Japs. This new bomb must be a son of a gun.

Thursday, August 15, 1945

Heard news of Japan's acceptance of our terms this morning at 8. First heard at 0100 hours this a.m. I should feel elated, etc., but honestly I don't—nobody here got very enthused. Only significant thing—it might get us home faster. No more dope on leaving except Pappy's rumor and I'm afraid of that one.

Friday, August 24, 1945

Orders came in today for 68 of us to leave here on the 27th as casuals. 5th Army stated that the probability was good that we'd go by air all the way. Knowing the army and how they treat the medics, I'm sure that won't happen. I'm happy because at least I'm now on the way.

Sunday, August 26, 1945

I'm down to a mere 65 pounds of baggage—just in case we fly. Sold my radio, trench coat, etc. We leave here at 6 a.m. tomorrow to go to Verona airport—its three hours from there to Naples by air.

Monday, August 27, 1945

We're staying with the 37th General Hospital tonight about half an hour from the airport. When we got to the post this a.m., we found that some general needed our four planes for a special mission in Austria. Fortunately, we didn't have to go back to Riva. We're promised the same planes for tomorrow—we'll see.

Tuesday, August 28, 1945

Left Verona at 9:25 and arrived Naples at 11:30. Beautiful day for flying and so we flew in a straight line over some of the most rugged country you'd ever care to see. (C-47s carried us—four of them.) Had lunch at the airport (place is littered with combat planes—now useless) and then were driven (in trucks as usual) to the 539th Company 29th Battalion of the 7th Replacement Depot out at the fairgrounds. As things stand now, we're no longer a group—just a collection of casuals and, what's more, M.D.s frequently go through more slowly than others. Filled out lots of papers with still more for tomorrow.

Thursday, August 30, 1945

Just back from a day at Pompeii. Bob W. [probably Wylie] had never seen it so I hitched out with him. We took pictures galore. It was a hot, dirty, dusty trip and I'm dead. Back here at 8:00 to find that all casuals are frozen. The *Mt. Vernon,* a naval transport, is in, so maybe some of us might make it.

Friday, August 31, 1945

If this goes on much longer I'm afraid the army will have a bunch of psychos on its hands. We're still frozen but nothing seems to be happening. Few officers leaving from the other billet, but none from ours.

Saw the first reel of a movie tonight but it stunk so that we had to leave—Billie Burke should give up.

Thursday, September 6, 1945

That great day—orders for home by air. In a week or maybe less I'll be with my wonderful family again. It's so good I can hardly believe it.

Spent the day at the beach, then to the Giardino degli Aranica for dinner—back here at 9 to find the orders on the board. 13 of us leaving by the "green plan"[5]—rest follow in next few days. We fly from here to Casablanca—B-17s, then by A.T.C. [Air Transport Command] in C-54s to the States—oh, am I happy.

Friday, September 7, 1945

A thousand good-byes at the annex to my friends in the aux. (Probably will see some of them in Casa.) Tonight we're held in the Caserna downtown in Naples—an old Italian fort overlooking the Bay of Naples. About 200 enlisted men and 20-some officers. We're leaving at 8:30 for Casa by B-17s. My last night in Italy.

Saturday, September 8, 1945

Casablanca again. Left Naples at 8:30 a.m. Just as we got out over the Bay of Naples the automatic life raft ejector threw a life raft out. It hit the plane just where I was sitting and I thought I was shot. We had to turn back to pick up a new one.

Instead, we took a new ship and then took off again at 10 of 10. Had a very uneventful trip—touched southern tip of Sardinia, flew over Naples and Oran, and landed in Casa at 4:45. We're billeted in Camp Dushane tonight and may be here up to two days. Fairly nice setup (tents) but well fixed—lots of bougainvillea out—very colorful.

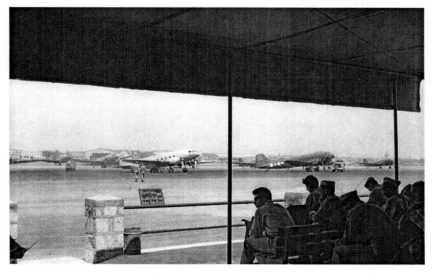

In limbo at the Naples airfield

Sunday, September 9, 1945

Mass at 9:00. Spent the day just waiting but nothing appeared on the board. In my tent there's a flyer who just came in from the States—he's on his way to Burma. Two other fellows in the tent are westbound from India. This little piece of world seems to be an international crossroads. We're confined to the post so I can't get into Casablanca. I guess I saw enough of it a few years ago.

Monday, September 10, 1945

Still in Casa. Supposedly the Green Project ended as of midnight tonight, so now we're supposed to fly more directly—Azores, Bermuda, then Florida. They had been going to Dakar, Ascension, Natal, then up. We're wasting lots of good weather just sitting here, but there's nothing you can do about it but wait.

Wednesday, September 12, 1945

They're hitting all around us but I'm still here. Lyman Brewer left this afternoon at 4, so we should be on our way pretty soon. Weather still good but I'm afraid it won't hold out 'til I get going. Absolutely nothing to do here and it's enough to drive a fellow crazy.

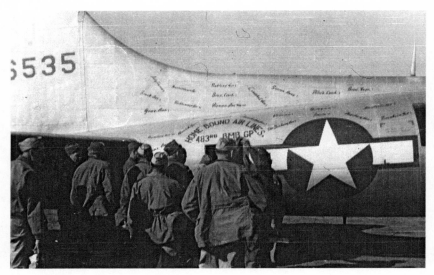

"Home-Bound Airlines," Casablanca

Friday, September 14, 1945

Bermuda.

We got notice yesterday noon that we were to leave Casa at 6 p.m. Took me just two minutes to pack. Drove through the city on the way to the airport and this was my last look at anything so foreign. Ours was flight 966, plane #9124, a C-54 and a plush seat-job at that. Really a beautiful piece of airplane and although an ocean hop is not something to be taken lightly, I felt confident that this ship could take us home safely. Left Casa at 1812 hours. We immediately got above the clouds out of a dreary day into brilliant sunshine. It was like having a fluffy quilt below us. The weather was perfect all the way to the Azores. It was dark when we pulled into Santa Maria and, although there were a few rain clouds, we could see the field—the runway lit up like a long narrow pathway. Landed at 2344 hours G.M.T. Had a supper there and then, after dropping two passengers so as to take on extra gas, we took off at 0170 hours G.M.T. We took off without mishap—I slept off and on through what seemed to be a very long night. I took a Seconal tablet to help me sleep—and it was a help. Dawn revealed a million small clouds below us and down beneath them a very blue and surprisingly calm ocean. Bermuda came into view just before 10:00 (Bermuda time). From the air it's a beautiful sight—a chain of islands in a green sea whose entire course is punctuated with white-roofed houses. It was a pleasant introduction to Bermuda. We landed at 1300 hours G.M.T. A W.A.C. [Women's Army Corps] lieutenant came on the plane and told us that we would have to stay overnight because a hurricane was threatening the Florida coast. If we had to be delayed, we couldn't have picked a better spot. We were billeted in the DeSink (A.T.C.'s hotel deluxe)—all other officers were put up in the wooden barracks for transients—why we're here is a mystery but it's a beautiful spot. Took off for Hamilton (capital of Bermuda) in the afternoon and had a good steak dinner there at the Ace of Clubs. Had a real malted milk shake earlier in the afternoon. Sent a cable to Marion.

Sunday, September 16, 1945
Still in Bermuda with no promise that we'll be out of here soon. Radio says the storm is heading northeast. Hot as all blazes here. Swam this afternoon.

Monday, September 17, 1945
Called out of bed at quarter of 7 this morning—planes started taking off at 4:30 and somehow we were overlooked 'til the last moment. Didn't have time for breakfast but rushed to the plane. Took off at 0731 Bermuda time. Weather perfect again and ride was a real pleasure.

Had coffee and a K ration breakfast. Flew over the Bahamas, then to Miami. Landed at 11:59 Florida time. Miami hot as the devil and you're continually wet with perspiration. Several thousand came in here by air this morning and they're set up to take care of only a small part of that number—consequently things are unpleasant. We're scheduled to go to Camp Blanding tomorrow night.

The big thrill of the day was talking to Marion. As soon as I got in here I tried to call but there was a big line to sweat out—finally at about 3 I got through. Her voice sounded wonderful and I couldn't say the million things I planned. Now there's the time 'til I see her to sweat out.

Tuesday, September 18, 1945
Miami to Blanding. Leaving here at 7 for Blanding by troop train. Supposedly we'll only have a short stay there. This place has been a sad disappointment—a dog.

Wednesday, September 19, 1945
Blanding. Left Miami at 1907 hours last night and traveled by day coach (first one ever built) to this post. Arrived here at 0400 hours. Filthy dirty,

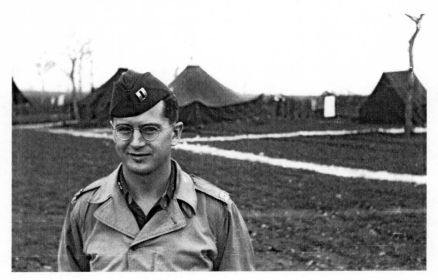

Captain Paul A. Kennedy, MD

hot, uncomfortable, tiring ride it was. Only bright spot was a 20-minute stop in West Palm Beach, where a local club had cold milk and cookies for us. Men and women, even small kids, came up to shake your hand and wish you a welcome home. It was a pleasant surprise. Hot here in Blanding but not as bad as Miami. We're leaving here this afternoon for Indiantown Gap, where I'll get out.

Epilogue

Get out he did—and went on to a long and successful career in private practice, first on his own in Buffalo and then in partnership with his Second Aux colleague Gordon Madding in the San Francisco Bay Area. The move to California was precipitated in part by the fact that my father's solo practice in Buffalo was too successful. He was no less dedicated to his private patients than he had been to soldiers on the battlefields of western Europe. Consequently, he was out of the house early and back late virtually every day. While satisfying, private practice also proved to be exhausting and stressful. Partnership with Gordon Madding offered relief. In fact, my mother believed that the move would add ten years to his life.

Ironically, then, the last years of my father's life were dismal. He was diagnosed with Parkinson's disease in the early 1980s, forcing his immediate retirement. He would live until 1993, increasingly disabled and increasingly demented.

When he could still speak but was becoming more and more confused, he would occasionally look at my mother and say, "I want to go home." She thought he meant their previous house, which he had loved and which they had to sell when he could no longer negotiate the stairs. I'm not so sure. Instead, I'm afraid that in the fog of his disease, he believed himself back in those miserable, homesick years of war and that in the end, not only did he lose his physical and mental capacities, he lost his home again, and this time forever.

Still, nothing could break his bond with his beloved Marion. In abso-

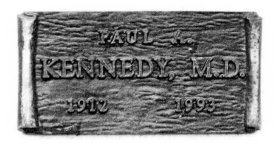

lute devotion, our mother cared for him at home every day—year after year—a bitter, heartbreaking duty, as the Paul Kennedy who loved her so fiercely slipped away, gradually but relentlessly. Through all those years she took care of him by herself. To the end. To the end.

Afterword

When Chris Kennedy asked me to read the manuscript of his father's World War II diary and then to write an afterword for it, I was reminded of the many great contributions that surgeons like Dr. Paul A. Kennedy made to the US Army during World War II. Their almost unceasing and prodigious efforts in the often dangerous and usually harsh conditions at the army's frontline medical facilities were crucial to saving the lives of thousands of seriously wounded and injured American and enemy soldiers and returning them to their families and useful lives.

I was most impressed with Paul Kennedy's diary because he had made no effort to rewrite it in the years after the war. Thus, as it is published today, it is little changed from the words that he first put to paper during those difficult days. He is exceptionally personal in showing his devotion to his Catholic faith and his deep love and longing for his wife and children. His thorough professionalism is revealed in the detailed case histories of his many surgeries and the post-operative care of his patients. A keen observer of what is going on around him, he provides numerous details on his travels, colleagues, and wartime experiences. Despite his best efforts and those of his surgical team, his surgeries of often horribly wounded soldiers were not always successful. However, it is obvious from his diary that each case provided him with a most important learning experience that he would carry into his long postwar surgical career.

Fortunately for the reader, Kennedy was also as ardent a photographer as he was a diarist. Many of the photos he took during the war now perfectly complement his diary entries and provide the reader with a graphic personal perspective, which is often missing from similar published works as well as from "official" US Army histories. His photographs do much to enhance the overall value of Kennedy's diary.

The medical unit in which Paul Kennedy served, the Second Auxiliary Surgical Group, was a most remarkable organization. Six of these groups were formed during the war and served in North Africa, Italy, France, and Germany. The Office of the Surgeon General, US Army, created these groups at the beginning of the war to provide expert surgical and postoperative care for American soldiers seriously wounded on the battlefield. These teams usually augmented the surgical and medical personnel of the field hospitals and divisional medical units, which generally lacked such skilled surgeons. They were constantly moved so that their skills could be brought to the aid of their Army Medical Department colleagues where they were most needed. The Surgical Consultants Division in the Surgeon General's Office carefully selected the most highly qualified and best-trained young surgeons to fill out the specialty surgical teams that made up the auxiliary surgical groups. The distinguished civilian surgeons now on active duty in the Surgical Consultants Division realized the enormous physical and emotional burdens that these front-line surgeons would have to carry day in and day out, often for seemingly endless hours at a time, and that particular requirement put a premium on youth. Paul Kennedy's diary very clearly shows the great strains their surgical workloads placed on these doctors, who often were moved to support field hospitals and divisional surgeons during periods of peak combat in Italy, France, and Germany.

In March 2000, when I was the chief historian for the Office of the Surgeon General, US Army, and the US Army Medical Command, I had the great privilege of meeting and interviewing Dr. Michael E. DeBakey, the renowned surgeon and pioneering heart surgeon. Dr. DeBakey joined the Surgical Consultants Division at the Surgeon General's Office in 1942 and was deeply involved with the selection and training of the surgical personnel of the auxiliary surgical groups before their deployment overseas. During the war DeBakey also made frequent extended trips to combat zones in the Mediterranean and Europe to review surgical procedures and the work of the surgeons in order to develop a set of uniform practices in the care and treatment of battle casualties throughout the Army Medical Department. When Paul Kennedy met DeBakey—during the selection process, during the war, or after the war—we do not know, but we do know from Chris Kennedy that his father definitely knew DeBakey.

During my interview with Dr. DeBakey, I asked him about the importance of the wartime experiences of these young surgeons, such as Paul Kennedy, to their postwar civilian careers. He told me how invaluable this experience was not only for the individual surgeons themselves but also for the postwar development and blossoming of American surgery and medicine. DeBakey noted that a surgeon in civilian practice would normally not experience in a year the volume and severity of traumatic wounds and injury that auxiliary surgical group surgeons often dealt with in a single day during heavy combat operations. He believed that this enormous learning experience significantly enhanced the quality of postwar medical school education and training as well as residencies in the specialty surgical fields: many of these surgeons returned from the war to assume clinical positions in medical schools and teaching hospitals and thus were able to pass along the many things they had learned under great stress in the battlefield hospitals. Paul Kennedy's wartime diary and subsequent long surgical career, both as a clinical professor of surgery and in private practice, certainly provide ample proof of the validity of Dr. DeBakey's contention.

One of the aspects of the history of the Second Auxiliary Surgical Group was its meticulous collection of medical and surgical data on its thousands of cases. The Second's commanding officer, Colonel James H. Forsee, Medical Corps, insisted that during their rather infrequent periods of rest his surgeons complete full clinical records of their surgeries for use in later research and publications. Paul Kennedy personally kept such case records of his surgeries, but he was not pleased that while he was enjoying occupation duty in June 1945 Colonel Forsee assigned him the task of compiling all of the charts and graphs, as well as contributing many of his personal photographs, to the Second's records into the large, two-volume report on its wartime activities that was to become *Forward Surgery of the Severely Wounded: A History of the Activities of the 2nd Auxiliary Surgical Group, 1942–45*. This extensive collection became the basis for *General Surgery,* published in 1955 as volume 2 of the Surgery in World War II subseries of the US Army Medical Department's official World War II history that Dr. DeBakey edited. Paul Kennedy, along with his wartime colleagues Gordon Madding and Knowles Lawrence, contributed chapter 21: "Wounds of the Liver and of the Extraphepatic Biliary Tract (829 Casualties)" to this work.

When Dr. DeBakey and the Surgical Consultants Division devised the concept for a new surgical hospital for the US Army in 1945, they based it heavily on the experiences of the auxiliary surgical groups and their surgical teams, such as Paul Kennedy's, in the Mediterranean and European theaters. That new hospital was called a mobile army surgical hospital, or MASH. Provided with its own organic transportation and hospital equipment so it could easily move from one location on the battlefield to another as required, the MASH could be in full operation within mere hours. From their first appearance after World War II until the last one was inactivated in October 2006, the army's MASH units established an unrivaled record in saving the lives of thousands upon thousands of American and enemy combatants as well as civilians in theaters of active combat operations around the world. Thanks to Dr. Paul A. Kennedy and to Chris Kennedy, who has generously shared his father's diary, we now have an intimate and dramatic view into the experiences, thoughts, and emotions of an army surgeon who not only saved hundreds of wounded soldiers during the war but whose labors and achievements also helped to pioneer an organization that saved many thousands more in later years.

John T. Greenwood, PhD
Former Chief Historian
Office of the Surgeon General,
US Army/US Army Medical Command

Acknowledgments

You could say that this book was seventy years in the writing, from the day of my father's final diary entry until its publication more than twenty years after his death. My own small part in it, in fact, didn't begin until after he died, when my mother shared with me his diaries and medical journals, of which I had been unaware up to that point. So my first thanks are to her—now more than ten years in the grave alongside my father—who not only started me on this project but made the first pass at editing the diaries. But of course my gratitude to her—the incomparable Marion—extends far, far beyond the narrow confines of this undertaking. She was in part responsible for my love of literature, of writing, of scholarship. Our parents conferred great gifts upon all of us siblings, and the greatest were the intangibles that have long survived the material necessities they also provided.

Thanks also to my four "older" sisters—Joan, Ruth, Deirdre, and Kelly—whose interest and support have been invaluable and whose love and concern for their brother have been sustaining forces. My children—no longer children now—my son, Joe, and my daughter, Marion, and her husband, Bryan Amos, were unfailingly encouraging, even after reading early rough versions of this manuscript.

I am grateful to Jack Kimel, who also read an early copy (and who is convinced that he is related to the Kimel family mentioned early in the diary), for perceptive and useful suggestions. Thanks to Sue Harnett as well, for guidance in the process of digitizing more than fifteen hundred photographic negatives.

An old friend, Eric Shinseki, made the resources of the Veterans Administration available as I attempted to track down Dad's surviving patients. In this effort, David Newman of the VA provided enthusiastic and effective assistance. He found three surviving vets who were willing—even, in one case, eager—to talk to me about their experiences. That he couldn't find more was my fault. By the time I had the idea, it was too late; most of them had died.

Roger Cirillo of the Association of the United States Army was committed to this project from the start and guided me through the early stages of publication. He also secured the thoroughly knowledgeable John Greenwood as an early reader of the manuscript. John's suggestions for the improvement of the text were absolutely invaluable, as is the afterword he graciously agreed to write. Allison Webster of the University Press of Kentucky was unfailingly, enthusiastically, and cheerfully helpful throughout the final year on the road to publication. If you set out to design the ideal copy editor, you'd wind up with Robin DuBlanc; she made the editing process a pleasure and immeasurably improved the final product.

In providing historical context for many of Dad's diary entries, which were sometimes elliptical or allusive, I consulted a number of excellent histories, none more helpful than Rick Atkinson's Liberation Trilogy. This was true in part because the three volumes trace almost exactly Dad's path through North Africa, Italy, France, and Germany but, more important, because they are exhaustively researched, authoritative, and compellingly readable. Moreover, he took a personal interest in this project, was instrumental in advancing it to publication, and was generous enough to write a foreword. I will always be grateful for his assistance to a bumbling amateur. It was like being a ten-year-old again and getting a hitting lesson from Willie Mays.

My inexpressible gratitude to my father—always and in all things my hero—is all-encompassing. He was a great, great man.

Finally—my everlasting gratitude and love to my late wife, Ana, for all that was and now is not, but never to be lost.

Notes

Introduction

1. Cowdrey, *Fighting for Life*, 18, 19.
2. Ibid., 173.
3. Smith, *The Medical Department*, 145.
4. *Forward Surgery of the Severely Wounded: A History of the Activities of the 2nd Auxiliary Surgical Group, 1942–45*, 858. In citing this work, I am using the original 1945 typewritten report to the surgeon general, not the later published version.
5. Cosmas and Cowdrey, *The Medical Department*, 380.
6. Cowdrey, *Fighting for Life*, 161.
7. Churchill, "The Scope and Nature of Military Surgery," 148.
8. Cowdrey, *Fighting for Life*, 162–63.
9. *Forward Surgery*, 863, 866.
10. Ibid., 673.
11. Ibid., 880.
12. Section 6, General Order No. 39, Fifth Army Headquarters, April 9, 1945.

1. Operation Torch and North Africa

1. Robert W. Robertson, assistant general surgeon, October 2, 1942–April 5, 1943, and general surgeon, April 5, 1943–August 27, 1945.
2. Lawrence E. Hurt, general surgeon, September 22, 1942–February 8, 1945.
3. Reeve H. Betts, thoracic surgeon, September 22, 1942–August 27, 1945; Gordon F. Madding, general surgeon, September 22, 1942–August 27, 1945; Leigh K. Haynes, assistant general surgeon, October 10, 1942–March 16, 1945, general surgeon, March 16, 1945–March 31, 1945.
4. Victory mail: The military compressed mail onto microfilm and shipped the rolls to V-mail stations, where they were "blown up" and delivered to the recipients. One advantage of this system was that it saved considerable cargo space for war materials.
5. Bernard Bolton, assistant orthopedic surgeon, September 28, 1942–January 1, 1943.
6. Alexander F. Russell, general surgeon, September 28, 1942–February 22, 1944.

7. Fred J. Jarvis, general surgeon, September 22, 1942–March 26, 1945; Ralph A. Munslow, neurosurgeon, September 28, 1942–August 3, 1944.

8. Norris H. Frank, anesthetist, September 28, 1942–August 27, 1945.

9. Werner F. A. Hoeflich, anesthetist, October 2, 1942–August 27, 1945.

10. Daniel V. Dougherty, shock team, December 2, 1942–March 12, 1943.

11. Lawrence M. Shefts, thoracic surgeon, August 26, 1942–August 27, 1945.

12. Anthony J. Emmi, shock team, October 10, 1942–March 7, 1943, assistant general surgeon, March 7, 1943–August 27, 1945.

13. Harold L. Poole, general surgeon, September 24, 1942–August 27, 1945; Frederick W. Bowers, anesthetist, September 28, 1942–August 27, 1945; Charles E. Dowman, neurosurgeon, September 16, 1942–August 27, 1945; Lyman A. Brewer III, thoracic surgeon, September 17, 1942–August 27, 1945.

14. Amanda R. Campo, nurse, operating room, February 23, 1943–March 31, 1944; Benjamin I. Schneiderman, anesthetist, March 7, 1943–August 27, 1945; George A. Delorey, surgical technician, October 20, 1942–July 9, 1945; George W. Clark, surgical technician, October 20, 1942–August 27, 1945.

15. Herbert J. Brinker, general surgeon, September 28, 1942–February 5, 1945.

16. John E. Adams, orthopedic surgeon, September 26, 1942–January 31, 1944; George E. Donaghy, anesthetist, October 5, 1942–August 27, 1945.

17. After the war Francis Arthur Philip d'Abreu was consultant surgeon to Westminster Hospital in London and examiner in surgery at the University of London and the University of Cambridge. He was a contributor to Hamilton Bailey's *Emergency Medicine*.

18. Henry T. Ballantine, neurosurgeon, September 7, 1942–June 13, 1943, general surgeon, June 13, 1943–August 27, 1945.

19. Hugh F. Swingle, assistant general surgeon, October 5, 1942–March 7, 1943, general surgeon, March 7, 1943–August 27, 1945.

20. Atkinson, *The Day of Battle*, 221.

21. Keegan, *The Second World War*, 352.

22. Atkinson, *The Day of Battle*, 431.

23. William A. Weiss, anesthetist, September 18, 1942–March 20, 1944.

2. Southern Italy and Monte Cassino

1. Luther H. Wolff, general surgeon, October 5, 1942–August 27, 1945.

2. James M. Mason III, general surgeon, October 5, 1942–August 27, 1945; Lina J. Stratton, nurse, operating room, February 22, 1943–July 6, 1945.

3. Paul F. Hutchins, anesthetist, September 2, 1942–July 13, 1944, assistant orthopedic surgeon, July 13, 1944–October 8, 1944, assistant general surgeon, October 8, 1944–January 11, 1945.

4. Starting on January 5, 1944, he began to keep detailed and illustrated records of each case that he did, first as an assistant surgeon and then, begin-

ning in November 1944, as head of his own team. He numbered these cases consecutively.

5. Atkinson, *The Day of Battle*, 355.

6. Keegan, *The Second World War*, 357–58.

7. Weinberg, *A World at Arms*, 661.

8. Laura R. Hindman, nurse, operating room, February 22, 1943–March 2, 1945.

9. Trogler F. Adkins, assistant general surgeon, October 5, 1942–November 20, 1944, general surgeon, November 21, 1944–August 27, 1945.

10. Atkinson, *The Day of Battle*, 348.

11. Lila LaVerne Farquhar, nurse, operating room, February 23, 1943–February 10, 1944.

12. Wooster P. Giddings, assistant general surgeon, September 16, 1942–October 7, 1944, general surgeon, October 8, 1944–August 27, 1945.

13. Clyde E. Flood, assistant general surgeon, March 7, 1943–April 5, 1944.

14. Wolff, *Forward Surgeon*, 82.

15. Irwin Kaplan, anesthetist, March 2, 1944–August 14, 1945.

16. Beverly T. Towery, shock team, March 31, 1944–August 27, 1945.

17. Frank W. Hall, general surgeon, October 2, 1942–August 27, 1945.

3. Anzio and Rome

1. In the course of the Anzio campaign, one Second Aux nurse was killed and eleven officers, two nurses, and five enlisted men wounded.

2. Wolff, *Forward Surgeon*, 40–42.

3. Clarence R. Brott, assistant general surgeon, March 7, 1943–June 28, 1943, assistant orthopedic surgeon, June 29, 1943–May 8, 1944, assistant general surgeon, May 9, 1944–August 27, 1945.

4. Operation Dragoon and the Pursuit up the Valley of the Rhone

1. Shirer, *The Rise and Fall of the Third Reich*, 1387.

2. Ibid., 1388.

3. The Maquis were members of the French Resistance who conducted guerrilla warfare against the German occupiers. They were named for the thickets of southwest France, where most of the Maquis cells operated.

4. Forces françaises de l'intérieur, the recognized armed resistance. As the liberation of France proceeded, they were increasingly transformed from a guerrilla force to light infantry and absorbed into regular French forces.

5. "Les Poulets" (chickens) was the scornful name given to women who engaged in relationships with Germans during the occupation.

6. As a colonel, Albert Walton Kenner was chief medical officer for Torch

and Overlord. After his promotion to brigadier general, he became medical inspector for AFHQ and surgeon to NATOUSA.

7. General Surgery Team 26 was made up of Kennedy, surgeon; Clarence Brott, assistant surgeon; and Freeman F. Brown Jr., anesthetist, as well as a nurse and two corpsmen.

8. Donald B. Williams, assistant thoracic surgeon, March 16, 1944–November 1, 1944, thoracic surgeon, November 1, 1944–July 16, 1945.

9. Helen L. Lang, nurse, operating room, February 22, 1943–July 6, 1945.

10. This probably refers to "War Wounds of the Liver," written with Gordon Madding and Knowles B. Lawrence (assistant general surgeon). It appeared in *Forward Surgery of the Severely Wounded*. Together they published a number of clinical studies after the war, many of them arising from their surgical experience in the Second Aux. Probably the most important was their book *Trauma to the Liver*, first published in 1965 and reissued in a second edition in 1971.

11. The waist-length "Eisenhower jacket" became standard issue for US troops in late 1944.

12. Colonel Forsee's "very conservative temperament was at times completely out of tune with his high-spirited officers." Brewer, "The Contributions of the Second Auxiliary Surgical Group," 319.

5. Germany, the End of the War, and the Journey Home

1. DUKW was not an acronym: D meant that the vehicle was designed in 1942, U signified "utility," K indicated driven front wheels, and W designated powered rear axles.

2. Beevor, *The Second World War*, 751.

3. Atkinson, *The Guns at Last Light*, 613.

4. This was a technique for treating fractures of the femoral shaft first developed in 1939 by the German physician Gerhard Kuntscher and refined throughout World War II.

5. The Green Project transported military personnel from the ETO to the United States via air.

Medical Glossary

Amputation
  Callandar's: Amputation at the knee joint with long anterior and posterior skin flaps, the patella (kneecap) being removed to leave a forma for the end of the divided femur.
  Guillotine: Rapid amputation of a limb by a circular sweep of the knife and a cut of the saw, the entire cross-section being left open for dressing.
  Traumatic: Amputation by injury.
Anastomosis: The surgical formation of a passage between two normally distinct spaces or organs. Intestinal a. is the establishment of communication between two portions of the intestine, commonly used in trauma when a portion of the damaged intestine has to be excised.
Anesthesia, endotracheal: Anesthesia produced by introduction of a gaseous mixture through a tube inserted into the trachea.
Appendix vermiformis: A diverticulum of the cecum.
Arteriovenous aneurysm: The rupture simultaneously of an artery and a vein.
Artery: Any vessel carrying blood away from the heart.
  Carotid artery: Principal artery of the neck.
  Mesenteric artery, inferior and superior: Originating from the abdominal aorta, the inferior supplies the descending colon and the rectum; the superior supplies the small intestine and the proximal half of the colon.
  Radial artery: Originating from the brachial artery, supplies the forearm, the wrist, and the hand.
  Ulnar artery: Originating from the brachial artery, supplies the forearm, the wrist, and the hand.
Atropine: Alkaloid used to relax smooth muscles or to increase heart rate.

Cardia: General term for the heart or the region of the heart.
Cecum: The intestinal pouch into which open the ileum, the colon, and the appendix vermiformis.
Cholera: Acute, infectious disease marked by severe diarrhea, vomiting, dehydration, cramps, prostration, and suppression of urine. Caused by *Vibrio cholerae,* contained in discharge from the bowels and spread by means of drinking water. High mortality.
Colon: The large intestine.
  Ascending colon: The portion of the colon between the cecum and the right colic flexure.

249

Descending colon: The portion of the colon between the left colic flexure and the sigmoid colon.

Sigmoid colon: The portion of the colon, located in the pelvis, between the descending colon and the rectum.

Transverse colon: The portion of the colon that extends transversely across the upper part of the abdomen between the right and left colic flexures.

Colostomy: Surgical creation of a new opening of the colon on the surface of the body.

Compression paralysis: Paralysis caused by pressure on a nerve.

Costal: Pertaining to the ribs.

Costochondral: Pertaining to a rib and its cartilage.

Costophrenic: Pertaining to the ribs and diaphragmatic pleurae.

Cystostomy: Creation of an opening into the bladder.

Suprapubic cystostomy: Cystostomy situated above the pubic arch.

Debridement: Removal of foreign matter and dead tissue in and around a traumatic lesion.

Disarticulation: Detachment of an articulated structure, such as a joint.

Diverticulum: A pouch or sac.

Drain: Creation of a channel of exit or discharge from a wound.

Cigarette drain: A drain made by surrounding a strip of gauze with a protective covering.

Penrose cigarette drain: A cigarette drain consisting of a piece of rubber tubing through which gauze has been pulled.

Stab wound drain: Drain accomplished by making a small puncture wound at some distance from the surgical incision and bringing out the drain through this wound to prevent infection of the incision site.

Duodenum: First portion of the small intestine, extending from the pylorus to the jejunum.

Ephedrine: An alkaloid used to relieve bronchial spasm or as a central nervous system stimulant.

Epigastrium: The upper middle region of the abdomen.

Eye enucleation: The removal of the eyeball after the muscles and optic nerve have been severed.

Femur: The bone that extends from the pelvis to the knee; the largest and longest bone in the body.

Fibula: The smaller of the pair of bones of the lower leg, extending from the knee to the ankle.

Fluoroscope: Device used for examining deep structures by means of X-rays.

Fracture: A break or rupture in a bone.

Comminuted fracture: A fracture in which the bone is crushed or splintered.
Compound fracture: A fracture in which the skin is broken.

Hemorrhage: Profuse or copious bleeding.
Herniation: Abnormal protrusion of an organ or other body structure through a defect or natural opening in a covering membrane, muscle, or bone.
Humerus: The bone of the upper arm extending from the shoulder to the elbow.

Ileum: Final portion of the small intestine, extending from the jejunum to the cecum.
Ilium: Superior portion of the hip bone.
Inferior vena cava: The large vein that drains the lower extremities, the pelvic region, and the abdominal organs into the right atrium of the heart.
Inguinal region: Pertaining to the groin.
Ischium: The dorsal part of the hip bone.

Jejunum: Middle portion of the small intestine extending from the duodenum to the ileum.

Laparotomy: Surgical incision through the flank or, more generally, the abdomen at any point.

Malleolus, lateral: The round protuberance on the lateral surface of the ankle.
Mesocolon: The process of peritoneum by which the colon is attached to the posterior abdominal wall.
Morphine sulfate: The most active alkaloid of opium, used as a painkiller.

Nembutal: Trade name of phenobarbital; a sedative.
Nephrectomy: Removal of the kidney.
Nerves, median, radial, and ulnar: Control the function of the forearm, wrist, hand, and fingers.

Omentum: A fold of the peritoneum extending from the stomach to adjacent organs in the abdominal cavity.

Perineum: Pelvic floor. In a male, the space between the anus and the scrotum.
Peritoneum: The membrane lining the abdomino-pelvic wall and enclosing the viscera.
Peritonitis: Inflammation of the peritoneum.
Plasma: The fluid portion of the blood in which the corpuscles are suspended.
Pleurae: The two serous membranes that surround the lungs (the visceral pleura) and line the thoracic cavity (the parietal pleura).
Pouch: A pocket-like space or cavity.

Morison's pouch: A pouch of the peritoneum below the liver and to the right of the right kidney.
Pulmonary embolus: A clot or other obstruction in the lung.
Purulent: Consisting of or containing pus.
Pus: Inflammation product made up of cells and a thin fluid called *liquor puris*.
Pylorus: The aperture of the stomach through which stomach contents pass into the duodenum.

Radius: One of the two bones of the forearm connecting the elbow and the wrist.
Resection: Excision of a portion of an organ or structure.

Sacro-iliac: The joint or articulation between the sacrum and the ilium, at the base of the spine.
Sacrum: Triangular-shaped bone wedged dorsally between the two hip bones.
Seconal: Trade name of secobarbital; a sedative.
Shock: Acute peripheral circulatory failure due to derangement of circulatory control or loss of circulating fluid; brought about by injury.
Small intestine: The proximal portion of the intestine, consisting of the duodenum, the jejunum, and the ileum.
Sodium benzoate: A white, odorless powder, used chiefly as a test of liver function.
Sodium citrate: A white, crystalline salt, used as an antacid, a diuretic, an expectorant, and a sudorific. Also used as an anticoagulant in blood for transfusion.
Spleen: Large, gland-like, ductless organ situated in the upper part of the abdominal cavity on the left side.
Splenectomy: Removal of the spleen.
Splint: A rigid or flexible appliance for the fixation of displaced or movable parts.
 Thomas splint: A splint for removing the pressure from the knee by transferring it to the ischium and the perineum.
 Tobruk splint: An immobilizing plaster cast splint applied from foot to groin with skin traction tapes through openings in the plaster and connected with a Thomas splint. Developed in North Africa in World War II.
Sucking chest wound: Traumatic opening of the lungs that causes partial asphyxia with collapse.
Sulfanimilide: Chemical used as an antibacterial agent; forerunner of antibiotics.
Suture: A stitch or series of stitches made to join and secure the edges of a surgical or accidental wound.
 Continuous suture: Suture in which an uninterrupted length of material is used for a series of stitches.
 Interrupted suture: Suture in which each stitch is made with a separate piece of material threaded on a different needle.
 Mattress suture: Suture in which stitches are parallel to the wound edge, the suture material crossing under the wound edge from one side to the other.
 Retention suture: A reinforcing suture for abdominal wounds, utilizing excep-

tionally strong material and including a large amount of tissue in each stitch; intended to relieve pressure on the primary suture line.

Tetanus: An acute infectious disease.

Tetanus toxoid: Immunization to prevent tetanus.

Thoracotomy: Surgical incision into the wall of the chest.

Thorax: The chest.

Tibia: The larger of the pair of bones of the lower leg, connecting the knee and the ankle.

Tracheostomy: Surgical creation of an opening into the trachea through the neck, for insertion of a tube to allow the passage of air to the lungs.

Typhus: An infectious disease caused by *Rickettsia* and marked by malaise, severe headache, and sustained high fever.

Ulna: One of the two bones of the forearm, connecting the elbow and the wrist.

Umbilicus: The scar at the site of the attachment of the umbilical cord ("belly button").

Urticaria: A vascular reaction of the skin marked by smooth, elevated patches often attended by severe itching, sometimes caused by a reaction to drugs such as penicillin.

Vein: Any vessel carrying blood to the heart.

Whole blood: Blood from which none of the elements, such as corpuscles, have been removed.

Selected Bibliography

Agnew, L. R. C., et al., eds. *Dorland's Illustrated Medical Dictionary*, 24th ed. Philadelphia: W. B. Saunders, 1965.

Atkinson, Rick. *An Army at Dawn: The War in North Africa, 1942–1943*. New York: Henry Holt, 2002.

———. *The Day of Battle: The War in Sicily and Italy, 1943–1944*. New York: Henry Holt, 2007.

———. *The Guns at Last Light: The War in Western Europe, 1944–1945*. New York: Henry Holt, 2013.

Beevor, Anthony. *The Second World War*. New York: Little, Brown, 2012.

Brewer, Lyman A. "The Contributions of the Second Auxiliary Surgical Group to Military Surgery during World War II, with Special Reference to Thoracic Surgery." 2nd ASG Distinguished Lecture, Uniformed Services University of Health Sciences School of Medicine, April 3, 1981.

Caddick-Adams, Peter. *Monte Cassino: Ten Armies in Hell*. Oxford: Oxford University Press, 2013.

Christopher, Frederick, ed. *A Textbook of Surgery*. Philadelphia: W. B. Saunders, 1945.

Churchill, Edward D. "The Scope and Nature of Military Surgery." In *A Textbook of Surgery*, edited by Frederick Christopher. Philadelphia: W. B. Saunders, 1945.

———. *Surgeon to Soldiers*. Boston: J. B. Lippincott, 1972.

Clark, Lloyd. *Anzio: Italy and the Battle for Rome—1944*. New York: Grove Atlantic, 2006.

Cosmas, Graham A., and Albert E. Cowdrey. *The Medical Department: Medical Service in the European Theater of Operations*. Washington, DC: Center of Military History, 1992.

Cowdrey, Albert E. *Fighting for Life: American Military Medicine in World War II*. New York: Free Press, 1994.

Ellis, John. *On the Front Lines*. New York: John Wiley & Sons, 1991.

Gray, Henry. *Anatomy, Descriptive and Surgical*. Philadelphia: Running Press, 1974.

Groom, Winston. *1942: The Year That Tried Men's Souls*. New York: Grove Atlantic, 2005.

Hastings, Max. *Inferno: The World at War, 1939–1945*. New York: Vintage, 2012.

Keegan, John. *The Second World War*. New York: Penguin, 1989.

Kerner, John A. *Combat Medic: World War II.* New York: iBooks, 2002.

Kershaw, Alex. *The Liberator.* New York: Crown, 2012.

Kershaw, Ian. *The End: The Defiance and Destruction of Hitler's Germany, 1944–1945.* New York: Penguin, 2011.

Liddel-Hart, Basil. *History of the Second World War.* London: Weidenfeld Nicolson, 1970.

Orr, Thomas G. *Operations of General Surgery.* Philadelphia: W. B. Saunders, 1943.

Shirer, William L. *The Rise and Fall of the Third Reich.* New York: Fawcett Crest, 1960.

Smith, Clarence McKittrick. *The Medical Department: Hospitalization and Evacuation, Zone of the Interior.* Washington, DC: Center of Military History, 1989.

Weinberg, Gerhard L. *A World at Arms: A Global History of World War II.* New York: Cambridge University Press, 2005.

Wiltse, Charles M. *The Medical Department: Medical Service in the Mediterranean and Minor Theaters.* Washington, DC: Center of Military History, 1963.

Wolff, Luther H. *Forward Surgeon.* New York: Vantage, 1985.

Index

CPSIA information can be obtained at www.ICGtesting.com
Printed in the USA
BVOW05*1956150416

444252BV00003B/5/P

9 780813 167237